Enneagram of Healing

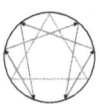

Also by Irv Givot

*Seven Aspects of Self Observation* (1998)
*Moments of Consciousness* (2001)
*Healing in China* (2004)

# Enneagram of Healing
## Exploring a Process

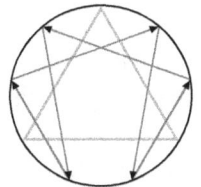

## Irv Givot

ATOM Press
Mercer Island, Washington

ATOM Press
2452 - 60th Ave SE
Mercer Island, WA 98040
www.accomplishtheimpossible.com

Copyright © 2012 by Irv Givot
All rights reserved. No part of this book may be reproduced or utilized in any form or by any means, electronic or mechanical, including photocopying, recording, or by any information storage and retrieval system, without permission in writing from the publisher or author.

ISBN 978-0-9842405-9-3

Library of Congress Control Number 2012933933
Library of Congress Subject Headings:
Healing, Enneagram, Spiritual perspectives, Transformation, Human Development, Medical, Spiritual, Prayer, Process, Gurdjieff

First Edition 1.0
Printed on acid-free paper
Diagrams and book design by ATOM Press
Cover line drawing from an inscription on the breast-plate of a tortoise shell estimated to be over 3000 years old, and residing at the China Medical University, Taichung, Taiwan.
Author painting by Winnie Givot
Author contact: dr.igivot@gmail.com

To my patients,
who have taught me much of what I understand about
healing.

# Contents

Introduction ..................................................... 3

## Chapter 1
The Dawning of the Healing Octave ........................ 15
    Points Zero, One and Two ............................... 15
    The 1→2 Interval ........................................ 21

## Chapter 2
The Mi-Fa Interval of 2→3→4 .............................. 29

## Chapter 3
Point Four ..................................................... 39

## Chapter 4
The 4→5 Interval ............................................. 47

## Chapter 5
Point Five and the 5→7 Interval ........................... 57
    The 5→7 interval ......................................... 61

## Chapter 6
Point Six and the 5→7 Inner Line .......................... 67

## Chapter 7
Point Seven .................................................... 75

## Chapter 8
The 7→8 interval .............................................. 85

## Chapter 9
Point Eight .................................................... 97

## Chapter 10
The 8→9 Interval, Point 9 and the Completion of the Octave......107

## Appendix
Complete Enneagram Symbols..................................................117

## Acknowledgments..................................................................123

## Bibliography..........................................................................125

## Index....................................................................................127

# Figures

Figure In-1, Enneagram Circle with Points Numbered ................... 7
Figure In-2, The Inner Lines of the Enneagram ............................. 9
Figure In-3, Enneagram Circle with the Triangle ........................... 11
Figure In-4, Enneagram Circle with Points and their Notes ............ 13
Figure 1-1, 0→1 and 1→2 Intervals and Inner Lines ..................... 25
Figure 2-1, The 2→3→4 Interval .................................................. 30
Figure 4-1, The 4→5 Interval and Inner Lines .............................. 54
Figure 6-1, The 5→6→7 Interval and Inner Lines ......................... 74
Figure 8-1, The 7→8 Interval ....................................................... 95
Figure 10-1, The 8→9 Interval ..................................................... 116
Figure Ap-1, Enneagram of Healing .............................................. 118
Figure Ap-2, Enneagram of Spiritual Development ....................... 119
Figure Ap-3, Enneagram of the Lord's Prayer ............................... 120
Figure Ap-4, Enneagram of the Transformation of Food ............... 121

The more we know about healing, the more we are carried simultaneously toward something unknowable.
For this reason, all healing is in essence, spiritual. Healing in the deepest sense is a mystery.
— *Richard Moss, M.D.*

# Introduction

This is a book about the process of healing—seen through the lens of the ancient symbol called the enneagram. The process of healing, as it unfolds through time, has much in common with the gradual awakening to the deeper reality within us, often called conscious evolution, or spiritual development. It is my hope that those with an interest in healing themselves or others, those with an interest in awakening to their inner reality, as well as those with an interest in the workings of the enneagram, may find valuable insights within these pages.

When one charts the steps of a process or a seven-aspected phenomenon onto an enneagram symbol—having some knowledge of the laws relating to octaves and triads—a whole new dimension opens up, and one can gaze into the process in question in an altogether different way, like looking at a drop of pond water through a microscope. New insights emerge, for example: seeing specific connections among the various steps of the process, understanding what difficulties to expect at different stages, and knowing where help is likely to occur. In other words, the effort to visualize a process graphically on this circular symbol yields results that are both enlightening and practical.

The process of healing is one in which I've had a personal interest most of my life; and from studying how it all comes together on the enneagram, I have learned a great deal more about the intricacies of this essential function in people. And surprisingly, my knowledge of healing gained over the last 35 years has made it possible to discover new subtleties of how the enneagram itself works. The enneagram teaches one about the process, and the process, if understood to a certain depth, can teach one about the enneagram.

Many years ago I made a first attempt to transpose the process of healing onto an enneagram symbol, trying mostly to identify and name the various points around the circle.

As I look back upon that early effort, I now realize that although it was imbued with the freshness and enthusiasm of trying to gain fluency in this new language I was learning—this deeper way of understanding the world—the effort came from the part of my mind that is used to solve puzzles or logical problems. In other words, my knowledge of the enneagram in the early 1980's was largely theoretical and borrowed from other students and teachers of the Work, and to compound the problem my understanding of healing, after only a few years in professional practice, was mostly undeveloped as well.

Now I am revisiting this effort 27 years later from a place in myself where there is not only more clarity about the fundamental cosmic laws embodied in the enneagram, but with more breadth and depth of experience relating to the nature of healing, on different levels. And what is also new is a trust in my own creative ability to visualize the essence of each gravity-center of the enneagram without reference to other authorities. The only exception to the latter, of course, is a continuing attempt to fathom the gist of the original formulations of George Gurdjieff himself. Because he was the one who introduced the enneagram to the Western World (c.1913), Gurdjieff's writings provide a frame of reference for understanding its workings and its applications. For that reason, and because of my own familiarity with both his teaching and his life experience, there will be many references to these in the ensuing pages.

The healing journey is intimately woven into my own path in this lifetime, both as a doctor practicing alternative/natural medicine, observing the many aspects and stages of healing and the inner attitudes and psychological changes that invariably accompany these stages in my patients, and also as a patient myself who has been attempting to heal himself from a chronic asthmatic condition with sometimes greater and sometimes lesser success for the last 60 plus years.

Because I have not yet completed my own healing, that is, reached a higher, more consistent level of health, there are many unanswered questions especially relating to the final stages of the process, that are motivating me to explore this process further.

On another note, it is useful to keep in mind that healing and health are derived from the same root as the word "whole." To be made healthy is to be made whole, and this can only happen in a strict sense when I bring all the parts of myself together, when I re-member myself. It is a matter of bringing a process that has been proceeding relatively unnoticed and in sleep—or else a process that is not proceeding at all because one has lost their way—more and more into consciousness.

Being conscious of the process is important for any person involved in healing himself or herself, so that they know where they are along the octave at each moment, and can thus understand the effort apropos to that stage. Also, being conscious of the process enables one's perspective to encompass the underlying laws of nature, including the relationships among the various steps conveyed in the inner lines of the enneagram. When a deeper understanding can emerge from a more conscious journey through the healing process then, as the saying goes, "The illness becomes the teacher."

One obstacle in the formulation in this enneagram is that healing is a big and wide subject, happens on many levels, and includes many distinct processes, that is, different octaves. Imbalances can occur at the molecular level, the cellular, the level of the tissues, organs, systems, the physical body as a whole, and also the psychological and emotional realms. These levels can affect each other in a complex labyrinth of interactions. I use the term labyrinth because most of these functions happen in a subconscious space not accessible to our ordinary experience or perceptions, except indirectly. In fact, people have widely differing abilities to tune into their body's inner workings.

In addition to the possible sources of imbalances in one's health listed above there are also the influences of what is called spirit or soul, which in turn are affected by one's past history, karma, and cosmic perturbations. Add to this the effect of the immediate environment around the person trying to recover, which often is a huge factor, and add further the process that the doctor or therapist themselves go through, and we can see that there are several different octaves that can be considered, and it is remarkably easy to confuse one octave, that is, one individual process, with another.

For this reason, I need to be clear that the enneagram of healing that we will explore here is the "patient's" octave, independent of the nature of the illness, injury, dysfunction, or whatever, and also independent of its cause, as well as the type of treatment rendered. Hopefully, this enneagram will be general enough to describe the healing of any imbalance on any level, although we are mainly interested in those abnormalities of function where one's own innate healing mechanism can't correct the problem in its automatic way. For example our bodies would heal a minor cut on the finger without the participation of our consciousness. In this study however, we are primarily considering imbalances where the body (or psyche) needs some kind of extra attention, either from oneself or others, or perhaps from a higher dimension of the universe, to enable the healing process. It is the nature of this "extra attention" that makes the healing process so interesting and such a challenge in real life.

However, even during the course of chronic conditions, our organisms are always attempting to heal in their own automatic, subconscious way. If we call all the healing influences pluses, and the stressful or toxic influences minuses, then it is simple arithmetic to see that if the pluses are greater than the minuses, healing can take place without our conscious participation but if (−) is more than (+) it means one's condition is going downhill and some kind of intervention is necessary for healing to take place—and it is this intervention that shapes the octave of our interest.

Another obstacle to the tidy formulation of healing in terms of an enneagram is that, especially in chronic conditions, rarely does one proceed from beginning to end—from onset to final resolution—in one smooth, linear process. There are fits and starts, repetitions of various steps, cycles within cycles, points at which people are stuck for years, and often there is the need to start over many times before the octave is completed, if ever.

So, facing reality, we must abandon all illusions of linearity. This octave, although it obeys the fundamental laws, is often very different from a one-time process with a definable clear end point, like preparing a meal. This non-linear quality of healing is one facet that makes it so interesting, but such a significant challenge to formulate with clarity.

In terms of the mechanics of enneagram formulation, there are two elements we are trying to understand at each stage of the process. The first element is the nine points or gravity-centers. These are distinct stages of the healing journey marked by an event, an experience common to that stage, or some obligatory shock provided by the cosmic laws, for every process, that enables the process to continue. These points are sometimes called "deflections." The process goes along in one direction and as a result of an experience or event marked by that point, the process changes direction slightly. In this sense, each gravity-center is a landmark for a transformation. The sum of all these changes of directions adds up to the approximation of a circle. (See Figure In-1)

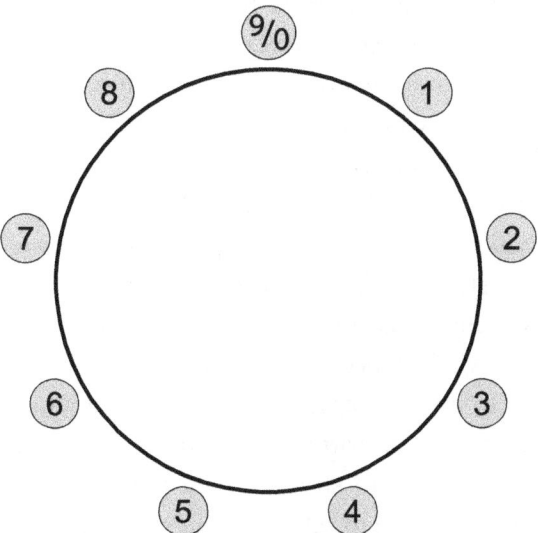

**Figure In-1,** *Enneagram Circle with Points Numbered*

Notice that we have adopted the convention of calling the beginning point of the octave, "0" and the point of completion, "9".

The underlying idea for the circle and the points is what Gurdjieff originally called the Law of Octaves, or the Law of Seven. An octave represents a doubling of vibrations—from the lower Do to the higher Do—and applies not only in music, but in all vibrational phenomena. In fact, in any process, from its inception to its completion, there is something analogous to this doubling of vibrations that follows the Law of Octaves, and allows it to be graphically shown on an enneagram. In Gurdjieff's words,

> If we grasp its full meaning, the law of octaves gives us an entirely new explanation of the whole of life, of the progress and development of phenomena on all planes of the universe observed by us. [1]

I would advise the reader to read or review pp. 122-132 of *In Search of the Miraculous* for a full explanation of these ideas.

The second element relates to the intervals between each gravity-center. There is a hint of mystery here. How does Do advance to or become Re? There is an apparent answer and beneath this, there is an abyss of unanswered questions, which I will leave to the reader to ponder.

These intervals, or as Gurdjieff called them, "stopinders", can represent (as I discovered while pondering the healing octave) a particular effort that is required to pass from one point to the next. This is part of what makes this study so informative and useful in a practical sense. In other words, being conscious of the appropriate efforts at each step will facilitate the whole process. Likewise, there are pitfalls or negative attitudes counter to each of these efforts at every stopinder, that are also totally characteristic of that part of the journey. Being conscious of these pitfalls can empower one to struggle with their demons at the precise moment when they threaten to sabotage one's progress.

In addition to these two elements, the gravity-centers and the stopinders (which are also called the points and the intervals, respectively), there are two further considerations at each point on the enneagram. The first is the inner lines, that is the connections between points 1 – 4 – 2 – 8 – 5 – 7, which represent relationships between two points and therefore

---
1 Ouspensky, P.D. *In Search of the Miraculous*, p.126

between the two experiences relating to these points. These relationships are like insights or visions or premonitions, or else reversions to previous stages of the process—that happen instantaneously or outside of linear time. It is incredible to realize that when we have certain key experiences in the context of this or any octave, assuming we are fully engaged in the process, we become connected simultaneously to corresponding experiences or events either in the past or the future. (See Figure In-2)

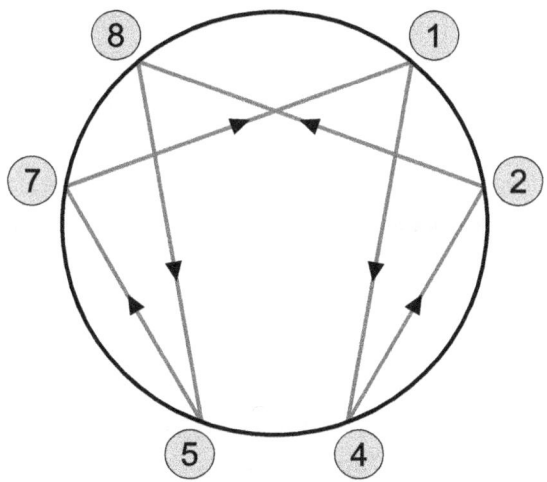

**Figure In-2,** *The Inner Lines of the Enneagram*

The inner lines are the connections between the successive numerals that result when 7 is divided into one. Seven divided by one yields the endlessly repeating decimal, 0.142857142857... The characteristic enneagram pattern inside the circle results from simply connecting the points 1-4-2-8-5-7 with lines between them. Each of these lines then, remarkably takes on a specific meaning in relationship to the whole process. Note that the inner lines 1→4, 2→8, and 5→7 advance forward, and thus when one is at point-one, two, or five in a process, there is the possibility of a vision to a future time when the process has come to these later points. Likewise, the inner lines 4→2, 7→1, and 8→5 look backward to an earlier stage of the process, so that when one is at point four, seven, or eight, an opening to reconnect with a past time in the process becomes possible, but there is a danger of reverting to the earlier stage as well.

The second additional consideration is the triangle of points 3, 6, and 9 which represents the Law of Three contacting the Law of Seven at the "shock-points", which Gurdjieff calls "mdnel-ins" (see Figure In-3).

The law of Three, like the Law of Seven, is another ancient formulation that Gurdjieff discovered that asserts that it requires three forces to produce a phenomenon. In modern times we are accustomed to thinking in terms of two opposing forces, like action and resistance, or male and female cells, etc., but to produce a phenomenon, or bring anything into creation, a third force is needed which is almost always very difficult to observe or identify. See pp. 77-79 of *In Search Of the Miraculous* for a more complete discussion of this "fundamental cosmic law."

Each place where one law affects the other causes a perturbation or shock that is necessary for the process to proceed. This is another deep mystery that I don't pretend to understand, except that we can describe the result of its action . By somewhat of an analogy, two of the fundamental physical forces, electromagnetism and gravity, seem to be almost totally independent of each other except that they coexist in the universe. None of the greatest minds of the last century had found a way to combine them into one more fundamental law of nature.[2] Yet these forces exist side by side and together determine the form and formation of the universe. The Law of Three and the Law of Seven are similar in this way, except for those definite points of interaction which allow the transformations that bring about the progress and completion of a process.

---

[2] That is, until the equations of string theory in the 1990's possibly accomplished this blending, but it is still unproven and somewhat speculative

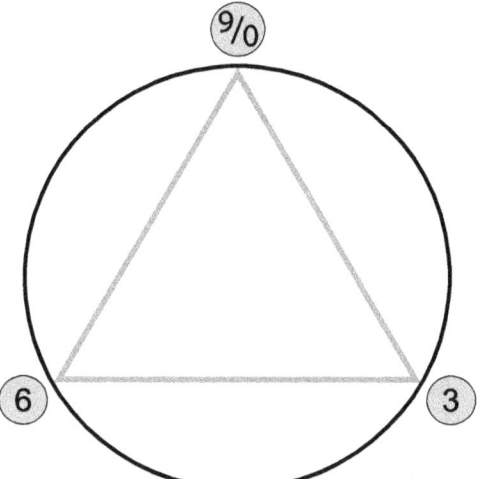

**Figure In-3,** *Enneagram Circle with the Triangle*

> The triangle represents the three forces acting on the process at these specific places. In the healing octave, at point-three the patient is passive, and the world is acting upon him/her. The patient becomes active at point-six, and the "world" is receptive. Point-nine is the neutralizing force in the triad.

There are some additional aspects of this inquiry that might be useful to briefly discuss, before we begin a detailed look at the actual enneagram of healing.

First, the aim here is to explore the nature of how a process unfolds and the laws that allow it to proceed, so that ultimately we may be able to understand ourselves and our world more deeply. An implicit aim, of course, is to find a way to actualize and complete the healing process both for myself as well as for the reader.

A process can be defined as a progression of transformations unfolding through time that leads to a higher level of order and some kind of completion, which then creates the conditions for a new beginning. Note that charting the progress of a process through time is a very different use of the enneagram than the popular application of studying personality types, or the listing of seven-aspected phenomena like the colors of the "white ray," the periodicity of chemical elements, and many others. These latter enneagrams help one to understand the characteristics of the types and see the relationships among them, etc. but there is no element of time involved, and no progression of a process. It is helpful to remember that the enneagram can be applied in all of these different ways, and one does not need to judge or declare either way to be more authentic or superior to the other.

Actually there is an enneagram in between the two poles described above and that is the octave of the days of the week. Although the progression of the days do not constitute a process in the sense I have defined, they do advance through time in a cyclic way, with a new beginning every Sunday morning; and each day has a unique character, like the nine personality types, especially for people who live according to a weekly schedule.

Another enneagram intermediate between those describing a process and those charting the seven aspects of a phenomenon is the enneagram of the notes of a musical octave. When an octave is sounded, not only is there a progression of notes through time, but there is an increase in vibrations with each one sounded, so that the higher Do has exactly twice the number of vibrations (also called cycles per second or hertz) as the lower Do (see Figure In-4). With electromagnetic waves, like light, a color with more vibrations (also called a higher frequency) has more energy, so that violet light has much more energy than red light. Likewise for the process of healing, as we progress toward health, the amount of energy available increases at each step. A healthy person has a lot more Qi, or vital energy, than a sick person, so we could say that robust health is a higher vibrational state than ill health. Like the notes of an octave plotted on an enneagram, each succeeding gravity-center of the healing enneagram represents a higher vibration than the earlier one.

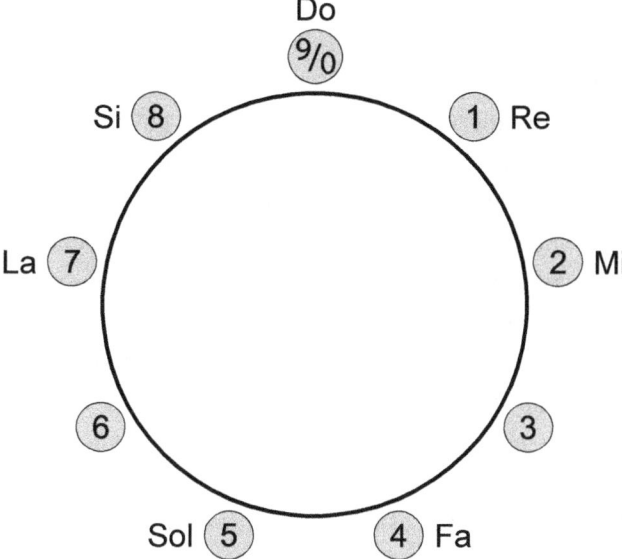

**Figure In-4,** *Enneagram Circle with the Points Numbered and their corresponding Notes*

> The notes are associated with the numbers representing the Law of Seven and the inner lines, with the exception of the Do, which occurs at the top of the triangle. This symbolizes the fact that the beginning and completion of a process are governed by a different law of nature than the rest of the process. This is another mystery to contemplate.

The enneagram of the musical octave has become a universal reference for enneagrams in general, so we may refer to the points around the circle by the note associated with that point as well as its number from time to time.

When several students of the enneagram try their hand at charting the same process—independent of each other—inevitably there will be different interpretations. In my opinion this does not mean that some are right and the others wrong, it simply shows that they have emphasized different aspects of the process, or are not really considering exactly the same octave. Just as there are an infinite number of points on a circle, there are probably a very large number of ways to describe a process.

And then there is the problem that those of us who are still students of the enneagram and not conscious masters, have the "blind men and the elephant" dilemma, where we are each able to perceive and elucidate particular parts, but nobody sees the whole in its entirety.

For this reason, I will beg the informed reader's indulgence and ask that you simply enjoy the anecdotes, stories, case histories, illustrative examples and small amount of theory that I will present, and suspend judgment, at least until the end, about whether the slightly unorthodox approach applied here, that goes beyond the standard method of enneagram interpretation, is a "correct" one. Then perhaps, like me, you may appreciate that the ideas and conclusions I have come to may not only advance our understanding of the nature of the healing process to a small degree, but that they may represent a new and fruitful way of understanding the workings of the enneagram itself.

## Chapter 1

# The Dawning of the Healing Octave

## Points Zero, One and Two

At the top of the circle is point-zero, the beginning, the Do of the octave. This point denotes the onset of an imbalance serious enough that the body's automatic functioning is not sufficient to bring about a spontaneous cure. For example, suppose one gradually develops pain in a shoulder. At first, the pain might not intrude into one's consciousness, except as a seemingly transient symptom that hopefully would go away by itself. The interval from point-zero to point-one represents the gradual awareness through time that there is a problem that is not going away. The culmination of this first step is the experience that marks point-one, which is the inner acknowledgment of this newly perceived dysfunction in the body. This unmistakable experience was immortalized in the story of *Apollo 13*, where after the explosion on the space capsule, the famous remark was communicated to the command station, "Houston, we have a problem." That is the essence of point-one: accepting that there is a problem that is not going away by itself, and recognizing the need for help.

The octave of healing, like that of many processes, starts at point-zero with what is called a "passive Do." It starts with a need, a lack of something, or in this case an imbalance in one's health—something that's not right. In general what sets the process into motion is the active response that occurs at point-one to that passive need.

In the case of the healing enneagram, the activity at point-one is a more or less intentional shift in one's attitude. As people often formulate it to themselves: "I have a problem, and I need some help." Most of us have had this kind of experience at some point in our lives.

As I noted in the introduction, part of the aim of this study is to become more conscious in real time of each stage of the healing process, that is, as one is going through it, living it, moment to moment and day to day. This includes an awareness of the obstacles at each step, which if they are observed, can be hurdled.

The most common obstacles to reaching point-one are denial and ignorance. These can be easily seen in certain types of people, for example addicts. In my practice, I have seen this happen to smokers, alcoholics, over-eaters, and those with a dependence upon other drugs, medications or even sugar. Point-zero is sounded in addicts when some threshold is reached—the physical body can no longer deal with the toxic burden and begins to break down, in some small way at first.

Ignorance during this stage means either not knowing that a symptom is significant, for example that an unexplained weight-loss or cough that won't go away might be a sign of cancer; or else ignorance in the Buddhist sense, that is, ignoring the problem, repressing it, not having the fortitude to face it. The extreme case of the latter is denial, where one actually deludes oneself that there is no problem at all, "I'm OK, there's nothing wrong with me."

A third weakness that prevents a person from arriving at point-one is procrastination, "I'll quit smoking (or other unhealthy habit) after the holidays."

Another category of people that are particularly susceptible to the obstacles at the 0→1 interval are the so-called type-A personalities. They are often so caught up in their careers, with all the stresses and demands on their time and energy, that they tend to tune out their bodies until the increasing intensity of the symptoms makes it no longer possible to do so. Then they react by making liberal use of pain pills, antacids, sleeping pills, etc. in order to sweep these annoying distractions out of their consciousness.

In my life I have known most of these obstacles first-hand. I have procrastinated seeking help; I have denied there was a significant problem;

I have ignored warning signs; I have taken drugs to cover up symptoms, and as a result there were a couple of times I almost didn't survive—which, by the way, are informative stories that I will include later.

The journey from point-zero to point-one can indeed have life or death implications. Some people die of massive heart attacks or strokes, for example, before they ever arrive at point-one, so that their final loss of consciousness just about coincides with the experience of the terror of their situation. Occasionally people die suddenly before they ever really cognized that they had a life-threatening problem at all. In these cases one might say that their healing octave was stillborn at point-zero.

On a more positive note, the ability to have a more or less conscious point-one experience can be a very important milestone. It is a turning point, and provides the impetus that sets the healing octave in motion.

The efforts that support the passage from 0→1 begin with inner sincerity: the willingness to impartially take an impression of the body's actual state, as much as one is able to perceive. This honesty with oneself can lead to the next effort, which is to have the courage to face the situation that one has glimpsed and begin to seek help.

A point-one experience that was pivotal for me happened around 1980 when, after a period of a couple of years of relative health, my asthmatic condition gradually returned, to the point where I could no longer control it with the methods that had worked before. This was during my early years at Two Rivers Farm, an intentional community where a large group of people were trying to learn and practice the teachings of Gurdjieff in rural Oregon. The help I received in this regard began by simply watching the other pupils. I noticed that on a few occasions when people revealed in group discussions the weaknesses they had observed in themselves, or the dark sides that they were struggling with, and simply asked for help in overcoming these obstacles from anyone present, in a sincere way that one could sense came from a place of real need, then they were literally showered with help and corresponding data from the others that felt inclined to speak. Over the course of time I was struck by the positive effects on those who were courageous enough to ask for help in this way, and I hoped that I would be able to find the inner strength to open myself also, when the need arose. So one week I took the risk and admitted that all the methods I thought I knew to help myself weren't working (including the usual asthma medications), that I needed help with my physical condition, and if anyone had any suggestions I would appreciate hearing them. Mostly I was asking about how to "be" with the problem, how to Work with it, rather than necessarily what to do about it. Several people responded and offered advice or related experiences of their own that were evoked by my request.

At the time of this writing, over thirty years later, I don't really remember any of the suggestions given that evening, but the lasting impression was the effect upon me of the admission of my helplessness. It was a breakthrough; it freed something in me from having to prop up the mask of invincibility—the old warrior archetype—which is an ancient, but now unnecessary trait of the male psyche. The irony is that in a close-knit community, the belief that one can hide their issues from other people is a delusion in itself.

Another conclusion that the above memory illustrates, is that there is a degree of healing that takes place at point-one, and as we shall see, at every point on the enneagram. When a person has a point-one experience, there is a release of pent-up tension from letting go of the irrational belief that one has to hide the problem from the world (and themselves), or be stoic and endure their (useless) suffering. At the same time, much energy is conserved from letting go of the fear of confronting and dealing with one's actual condition. There is some healing simply as a result of that act of inner sincerity.

Looking ahead, there is also healing that takes place at point-two, where the decision to embark on a specific course of action or a commitment to consult a particular doctor or therapist releases the anxiety and uncertainty that might build up on the 1→2 interval before the help one needs presents itself unequivocally. At point-four there is a tremendous relief when the treatment is finally underway.

But before we drift too far ahead of ourselves, there is another facet of point-one that needs to be mentioned. That is, this point is almost equivalent to the corresponding point-one in the enneagram of self-mastery, or spiritual development achieved by Work on oneself. In the latter enneagram, point-one is the observation and acknowledgment that something is missing from one's life and that something is not right in oneself. The acceptance of this can ignite one's search. An example is a story in *Beelzebub's Tales* about a legendary young man named Belcultassi who lived many thousands of years ago on the continent Atlantis, and was the one who discovered esoteric studies and the practice of Work on oneself. His discovery, which would effect humankind forever, started from this inner experience:

> When this .... Belcultassi was once contemplating, according to the practice of every normal being, and his thoughts were by association concentrated on himself, that is to say, on the sense and aim of his existence, he suddenly sensed and cognized that the process of the functioning of the whole of himself had until then proceeded not as it should have proceeded according to sane logic.
> 
> "This unexpected constatation shocked him so profoundly that thereafter he devoted the whole of himself exclusively to be able at any cost to unravel this and understand."[1]

However it is important to realize that this quality of commitment was only possible because of the depth of Belcultassi's observation of his life up to that point. In other words we cannot make a profound commitment just from self-will. The more we see about our condition—the way it actually is—the more sincere will be our decision to not only seek help, but to persist through the process until a real change is made.

The last sentence of Belcultassi's experience leads to point-two of the octave of self-mastery, where a total commitment was made to understand the "sense and aim of his existence" at any cost.

Likewise, in the octave of healing, if one can make this quality of commitment at point-two, the octave has a tremendously better chance of progressing to completion. In many ways the octave of Work on oneself (over a lifetime) is similar to the octave of healing, as we shall note as the discussion progresses.

One final aspect of point-one to discuss is the inner line from 1→4. This inner line can have different meanings in the healing octave since it occurs in another dimension of time and is thus more a part of our inner subjective experience than the measurable outer events that

---
1  G.I. Gurdjieff, *Beelzebub's Tales*, p.294-5

flow along the circle. Perhaps for people that have attained a higher level of consciousness, and are more fully engaged in the process, each inner line would have more of an objective nature. In fact one's experience of the inner lines may depend upon one's level of being or even upon one's attitude toward the process.

One meaning of the 1→4 inner line is as follows: as soon as a person has the experience of point-one—the definite acceptance that one needs help—it is as though one immediately receives a clairvoyant glimpse, a premonition, or a vision of what is to come at point-four. In practical terms it can be thought of as spontaneously looking ahead, visualizing, or anticipating the treatment or the form of help needed, so that one can follow that mental picture in actual life through the 1→2, and 2→3→4 intervals to make it really happen.

Sometimes this whole sequence can happen very fast, for example, in the case of a competitive athlete breaking a bone on a ball field. After he recovers from the shock in a minute or two, there is no way for him to avoid the point-one experience, especially if he tries to move and can't because of the overwhelming pain (this was a first-hand experience, by the way). At that moment the 1→4 inner line would be a visualization of getting the leg in a cast, as quickly as possible. One "sees" the treatment that is needed, but then has to live out all the preliminary steps.

Another example of the 1→4 inner line relates to the experience of certain patients of mine who suffer an injury or an onset of severe pain in some joint or muscle. Once they realize they need help, they sometimes spontaneously picture themselves lying on my treatment table, and receiving the adjustment needed to take the pain away.

On the other hand, there can be a negative aspect of the 1→4 inner line, and that is the dread or fear one can feel if they visualize a treatment that is particularly unappealing, and in their imagination would only intensify their suffering. This latter aspect of the 1→4 inner line is manifested in people with addiction or dependency issues who are afraid to trade the suffering of their newly perceived health condition for something they imagine might be worse. For example, when an alcoholic or smoker arrives at the point-one experience and has a glimpse of point-four, what they see might be that they must give up their habit in order to restore their health. If this is too frightening, the octave would hover in limbo somewhere between point-one and two. But a common secondary strategy to which addicts often resort is to continue to point-two but with the hope of finding a doctor who is willing to treat their new condition without demanding that they quit their habit.

For a doctor, this is a very difficult issue over which I myself have swung back and forth many times; but we need to remember that the doctor's quandary here is part of a different octave. In any case, for addicts of any kind, the premonition given by the 1→4 inner line could act as an obstacle to healing when there is the dread of some kind of loss, should the addicted person decide to seek help from an "unsympathetic" doctor.

For people whose symptoms may possibly suggest cancer—their dilemma involves looking ahead and visualizing standard medical treatments that may be more lethal than their tumor. These people may remain stuck at the 1→2 stage until it is too late, or else decide to search for less toxic experimental alternatives.

When a different category of people look ahead from point-one, what they see is the expense involved in embarking upon a certain course of treatment. This is the obstacle that stops many people from reaching point-two. Money problems are so entangled and intertwined with health care in our society these days that this has become an overwhelming problem for almost everyone unable or unwilling to pay huge medical bills.

It is so interesting that a glimpse into the future at point-one can be considered a gift from above, a sort of grace; but the reality is that what we see can encompass the whole spectrum from an answer to a prayer, to a terrifying possibility to be avoided.

## The 1→2 Interval

Regardless of what is seen along the 1→4 inner line, the next step is to seek out some help. On the outer circle, the 1→2 interval represents a new direction, and there are efforts unique to this interval that facilitate this section of the journey. The goal is to reach point-two, the place where a decision is made about a course of action, and also in a deeper way—in the way of Belcultassi—a place where a deep commitment is made to see the process through to the end. To assist in arriving at this inner commitment, the first effort is to find the motivation to seek what is really needed, rather than opting metaphorically for an aspirin or a Band-Aid. That is a tall order and obviously easier to talk about than to actualize; but this step is necessary to complete the healing octave, or even to arrive at point-eight. One source of motivation is to access the need in oneself to be healthy, which can be very powerful if one succeeds in reconnecting with it. This need may relate to what Gurdjieff calls, in *Beelzebub's Tales*, the First Obligolnian Striving: "the striving to have... everything satisfying and really necessary for their planetary body."[2]

Striving is a more appropriate term for this effort than need; it conveys a sense of aspiration, or the effort to reach for something that is essential to life, but may not be so easy to find. But a striving is also something with which a person may be so out of touch, that its absence may explain why the imbalance went as far as it did before the person woke up to it.

Occasionally the motivation to make a commitment to see the healing process through to its completion can come through one's wish to serve other people. In other words, the person may have precociously learned the value of putting others before oneself and understands that one must be healthy to work in that way. In the words of my former teacher, Mrs. Staveley, "to be of service, one must first be serviceable." This latter is a statement that is true on many levels. And the beginning of being serviceable is to be at least minimally healthy, otherwise it is next to impossible to be of service to anyone in any capacity.

There is some contention on that issue; a fellow pupil once observed that even a very ill person lying in bed may have insights into the cause of his illness that may be a help not only to the sufferer but to those around him or her. But on the other hand, consider that one of our functions here on the earth is to transform energy. Lower substances are transformed into higher ones, lower energies into higher energies. This is a possibility for a human being. And my experience is that when I am ill and struggling to breathe, what little energy I have is consumed by the struggle for relief, and no substantial transformation of energy, which in my understanding must be intentional, is able to take place. So when one is ill, very little of this more subtle type of service to the larger whole can be made to happen.

---
2  G.I. Gurdjieff, *Beelzebub's Tales*, p. 386.

The point is, that the wish to be of service can be a motivating factor to regain one's health, and thus be an encouragement to seek help in a timely fashion.

So far on the 1→2 interval we have mentioned motivation, striving, and wish as assets. These impulses are related to the heart, the emotional brain, but the use of the mind is also of practical benefit on this leg of the journey. If it is a worsening chronic ailment that brought the person to point-one, then they need to research the possibilities for various approaches to their healing. Sometimes there are many choices, or depending upon the dysfunction, only one or two. The skill of discernment is critically important at this step. If, for example, one hastily allows oneself to be coerced or intimidated into either submitting to a questionable surgical procedure, or agreeing to take a dangerous drug, prescribed by a less than competent doctor, the patient may regret it for many years or even for their whole life. If the treatment that begins at point-four turns out to be a fiasco, the patient must return to this point on the circle—the approach to point-two—to repeat that part of the process again.

So, making a wise decision at point-two is crucial, and as I have witnessed many times, the right-brain also plays a major role in this decision-making. With the left-brain one catalogs what is available and what seems to be the best choice, but then the right-brain performs its function, which is the use of one's instincts and intuition, and even prayer. A colleague related to me recently that a patient told him, "finding you was the answer to my prayers." In a similar vein, a man was driving along the street where I practiced, and as he related, his car seemed to drive itself into a parking space in front of my office, and he became a patient that day. Did he feel some energy even out on the street that was resonant with his need? Or was this someone who simply trusted some kind of subconscious guidance?

In any case, it is a question of focusing the mind and then connecting with the intuition. If one can really contact the higher centers in this way, one will receive what they need, often very quickly.

The main enemy of the 1→2 interval is fear. As we discussed earlier, fear can come into play when one looks ahead to point-four. Also laziness and procrastination for whatever reason, can prolong this phase by keeping people stuck in a treadmill of indecision.

✧

Point-two is reached when the decision is made fully and completely. It is also possible, as we discussed, to come to a deeper commitment to the whole healing process. Although the phrase, "whatever it takes," has been trivialized by overuse and has descended into a cliche in this period of time in which I am writing, there was a time a few years ago when that phrase was fresh, and it evoked an attitude of utter conviction that one would succeed in their aim no matter what difficulties appeared in the way.

I have felt this way a few times in my life. One example happened about 35 years ago when I decided to move to Portland from Colorado to attend Western States Chiropractic College. I could have easily been discouraged by the almost total lack of money available, by my weariness of going back to school yet once more, by again moving far away to a place that would be difficult for my hyper-sensitive lungs, and simply by the inertia preventing a major change. But when a decision is made from that essential place in oneself, there is an unstoppable force that can drive the process and overcome each obstacle as it arises.

Sometimes a new patient that I meet will have had a profound point-two experience and my response is delight, because I know their chance of recovery is strongly increased.

The gift that one receives at point-two when this note Mi is sounded with authority is a clearer vision afforded by the inner line projecting from point-two, the 2→8 inner line.

Point-eight for most people is the final step of the process, the place where their health is restored in a stable way. The inner line here shows one that choosing this path may lead them to this result. The 2→8 inner line is a preview of the first stable end-point of the process to which that particular treatment will lead. Figure 1-1 on the next page shows a graphic representation of this part of the enneagram. The complete enneagram of healing is shown in Figure Ap-1 on page 118 of the Appendix.

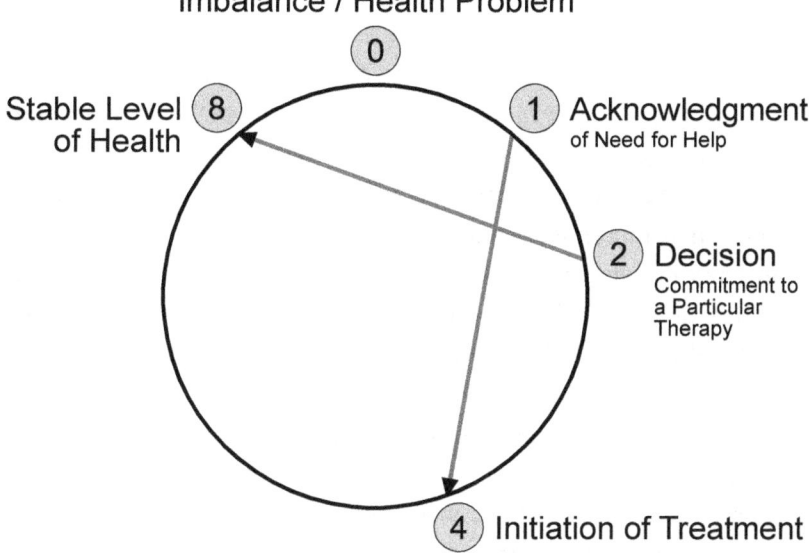

**Figure 1-1,** *Partial Enneagram focusing on the 0→1 and 1→2 Intervals and the associated Inner Lines*

> The 0→1 interval (the first stopinder) represents the growing awareness of the problem.
> During the 1→2 interval (the second stopinder) the person goes through a mini-process of deciding what to do about it.
> Once a person accepts the need for help, there is possible a visualization of the treatment needed (1→4 inner line), and once the decision is made about how to proceed, one receives a glimpse of the possible outcome of that decision (2→8 inner line). See Figure Ap-1 on page 118 in the Appendix for the complete enneagram of healing.

This preview (2→8) occurs exactly at the place where one makes a commitment to a specific path. Examples in other types of octaves: when an architect commits to a certain design for a building, he can then visualize the finished building. The same is true for an artist deciding to paint, for example, an impressionist landscape. Once a decision is made, then for a moment, the finished painting can be seen.

In the octave of the digestion and transformation of food in the human body, point-two is that part of the overall process where the digested food, in the small intestine, is broken down completely, and then absorbed into the body. (See "Figure Ap-4, Enneagram of the Transformation of Food" on page 121.) Only a certain fraction of the food can be absorbed from each meal so there must be a decision made by the "gastric brain" about which nutrients are most needed at that time. The 2→8 line here represents the ability of the innate intelligence of the body to see what nutrients are currently the limiting factors for the production of sperm and ova along with other cellular constituents and substances involved in the supporting metabolism. Survival of the species by reproduction is the overriding priority of one's automatic functioning. Point-two is where the commitment is made by the innate intelligence to carry it out—at least in that part of a woman's life between puberty and menopause and in a man's life from puberty until death, unless the impotence of infirmity eventually overtakes him.

However, the 2→8 inner line is also a way that we manifest that ability, unique to adults, to foresee the possible negative consequences of our actions. Sixteen year old boys, who often lack this ability, have the highest rate of fatalities driving cars compared to all other age groups and compared to girls of that age, because of that unfortunate combination of inexperience, adolescent hormones, and the inability to foresee the consequences of their decisions. When an older person has lived through a crash or two that could have killed them, they are more likely to visualize the possible outcome of a course of action, for example, a decision to drive a long distance on icy roads with a car that has substandard tires. Likewise, a patient with say, low-grade heart disease, can weigh and visualize the hazards of dangerous treatments, and may opt out of a particularly risky type of open-heart surgery based upon an intuitive feeling arising from the 2→8 premonition. Unfortunately many older adults often act like sixteen year-olds, not taking advantage of the 2→8 inner line, and sometimes rush headlong into the first treatment suggested to them.

In one sense, I feel that people (like me) who have had a chronic health problem are fortunate, because we have had the opportunity, over the course of many years, to learn how to manage it. When a new problem does arise for us later in life, we don't panic and aren't intimidated into accepting a drastic and dangerous treatment as the first option. I have seen too many seniors, who have been healthy all of their lives, and thus are totally naive about the medical system, who end up succumbing to the first serious health problem that befalls them. Interestingly there are always alternatives, and fortunately one can sometimes change course and find a new kind of treatment before it's too late.

The joke in parts of Mexico is that if a poor villager gets sick, he/she goes to the Shaman. If their treatment doesn't work the villager will travel to the city to consult a medical doctor. But if a wealthy urbanite gets sick, they first go to the M.D., and if that doctor can't provide the necessary help, then they will travel to the countryside to visit the Shaman.

## Chapter 2
# The Mi-Fa Interval of 2→3→4

The next step in the octave of healing, the 2→3→4 interval, also called the Mi-Fa interval, represents another change in direction, which entails a new kind of effort.

Once the decision is made at point-two, one needs to physically transport oneself to the doctor, hospital or wherever. Until now the process has all been internal. The movement from 0→1 and 1→2 occur within one's own experience, that is, within one's perceptions and impressions of the body and its travails, one's reaction to it, the acceptance of the need for help, the inner commitment to see the process through, and the decision to seek a specific form of help.

Suddenly, at the next stage, the approach to point-three, the rest of the universe becomes involved. The affected person proceeded up until that point with only their internal experience (and maybe the reactions from a small number of people with whom they shared it); now there is a collision with the outer world. This point is where the two cosmic laws intersect. A force from the external world meshes with one's internal process like the way gears do, and this coming together allows the person's octave to continue. Why the universe is this way is another cosmic mystery, but in practical terms, we can verify that the shock from the outer world occurs at this stage in every process. And in intuitive terms, it makes sense that at a certain early stage, the world must interact with one's intention, otherwise the process would remain internal and abstract, and could not proceed beyond this point; that is, there could be no further real transformation.

One can also visualize the interaction between the two laws (the Law of Seven and the Law of Three) as a triangle hovering over the enneagram symbol, that makes contact, like two live wires touching each other—first at point-three, next at point-six, and then at the approach to point-nine. Gurdjieff called the corner of the triangle that touches the enneagram circle at point-three, the "Mechano-coinciding mdnel-in." It is a mechanical shock coinciding with the nascent process, the point in time when one begins to manifest their decision in the material world. Here the two types of forces come together in a lawful way that enables the process to continue. (Figure 2-1 below illustrates this part of the enneagram.)

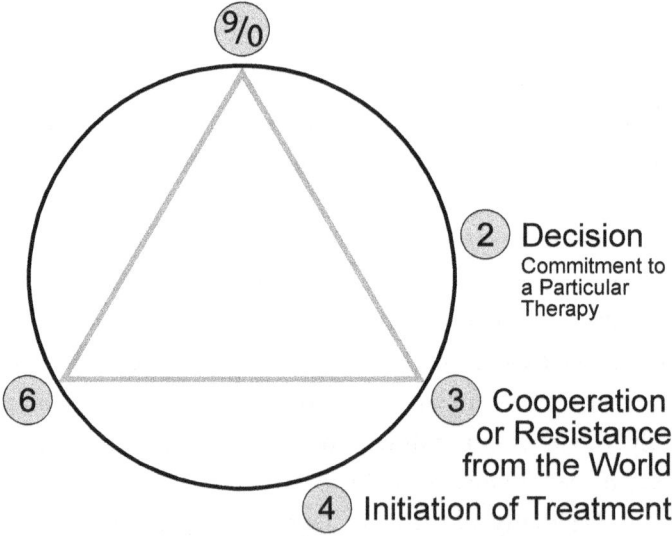

**Figure 2-1,** *Partial Enneagram showing the 2→3→4 Interval*

The 2→3→4 interval (the third stopinder, or mi-fa interval) is that part of the process where one attempts to actualize their decision, but must negotiate through the forces of the outer world (symbolized by point-3) in order to do so and reach point-4. Then one makes a material contact with the doctor, healer or therapy, which is in a way another beginning of the healing journey.

What "comes in" from the outer world at point-three, in terms of the healing octave, can be support or it can be resistance. For example, if one is seriously hurt in an auto accident on a snowy mountain pass, someone has to transport the injured person to a hospital. Outside help must come in to enable the healing process to proceed to point-four, where in this example, trauma care can begin in earnest. But the world can also be a resisting force. One can imagine many scenarios in which the injured person may not make it to the point of receiving the necessary help. The ambulance might get lost in the snowstorm and not find the victim in time. The ambulance might have an accident of its own, or a mechanical failure on its way down the mountain, etc., etc.

Consider another category of cases where a child needs immediate help, and an irresponsible or mentally disabled parent may deny the child medical intervention for a variety of spurious reasons, including religious belief systems, stoicism, perceived lack of resources, or simple neglect based upon denial.

Another example of resistance at this point involves women married to abusive or controlling husbands. I have seen many of these unfortunate women, whose husbands often refuse to allow their wives to even begin treatment in my clinic, again for a variety of strange reasons, including a disapproval of chiropractic, a (delusional) jealousy triggered by the thought of her being alone with another man, or the most popular excuse, usually articulated as, "we can't afford it." A wife who is fortunate enough to have a supportive husband, or vice-versa, or a child with caring and supportive parents, obviously have a tremendous advantage at this interval, this "shock-point."

In sum, in order to receive help, the world needs to cooperate. Often the "world" is the other people in one's life, but sometimes it can be more cosmic.

The other factor is that the strength of the person's resolve to find help may influence the outcome at this point. In other words, we may actually affect the triad of the "world" with the quality of our intention.

I once had a strong experience of the phenomenon that occurs at point-three, which was in effect the shock that started me on this journey into the profession of healing and also changed the direction of my life.

This seems like an appropriate place to relate that story. It was on New Year's morning of 1971 that I awoke in my apartment outside of Boston with an asthma attack severe enough that I knew I could not deal with it myself. When one is suddenly struggling for every breath, the point-one experience arrives rather automatically. In those earlier years of my life as a graduate student at Brandeis University, I had no concept of self-healing and no knowledge of natural alternatives to pharmacological drugs. The only real choice, given the urgency of my circumstances, was the emergency room at one of the big teaching hospitals in downtown Boston, twelve miles away, which I had already used six months earlier for a less severe attack. So, likewise, I arrived at point-two without hesitation. I simply told Winnie (my wife), "You need to take me to the hospital." She could see my distress and immediately went downstairs to get the car ready. I got dressed and struggled down the stairs from our third floor apartment, and staggered out into the winter morning. A heavy snow was falling; in fact it was almost a white-out, but otherwise peaceful and very quiet. I hurried out to the curb to get into the car that she had waiting. But by the time we were ready to go, as I sat hunched forward in the passenger seat of our tiny VW Bug, I was gasping for air. It was as though there was not enough air in the car. A panic reaction rose up in me and I impulsively jumped out of the car, and told Winnie to call an ambulance, as I began to feel the bizarre symptoms of oxygen deprivation. I staggered back up the hill to the front door of our building and collapsed in the foyer. As I laid there on the floor, unable to brush the snow off and gasping for every breath, a thought came to me from what seemed like a new place deep inside: "I might not make it." The next thought was, "I don't want to die here," then I lost consciousness.

I woke up about ten minutes later sitting in the back of a police car with an oxygen mask over my face. Ambulance service, for one reason or another, was unavailable that morning because of the heavy snowstorm, so a police unit was dispatched instead. The world arranged it so that I could survive. I'll never forget the look of intense concern on the face of the officer driving the patrol car when he turned to look back at me as I was regaining consciousness. It was one of those impressions that stays with one for their whole life. I could also feel the love coming from my wife, who was sitting right in front of me. Then I slipped back out of consciousness into what I later described as a "hallucinatory netherworld," where the predominate color was violet, or purple, and which was inhabited with strange entities who moved in illogical ways, but didn't seem to notice my presence at all. I woke up again when we arrived at the emergency room, and from that moment, my recovery, that is my journey from point-four to point-five, was uneventful and took about three days.

During that time in the hospital, and for many weeks afterward I was obsessed with the thoughts that came to me before I blacked out in the foyer of our apartment building: "I might not make it." After much pondering I realized that was the first time in my life I had seriously brushed up against my mortality, and in addition, it was the first time I had honestly faced my situation. Before that event, asthma had only been an annoyance and a nuisance in my life, and was something easily suppressed with pills when it began to interfere with vigorous activities. I never had a clue that for me this condition could be life-threatening, or that as an otherwise energetic and athletic young man, I would have to deal with my impending death in the foreseeable future. From my current perspective, to say "I faced my situation," was perhaps a self-deception because actually it was pointed out to me by a subconscious voice deep within that hitherto I had had no contact with at all (that I recall). But I did listen to it, and it made a deep enough impression that I remember it to this day. In fact, suddenly coming to a close encounter with premature death changed everything. I reevaluated all my priorities.

This reevaluation happens to many people who have lived through near-death experiences (more accurately, after-death experiences). People that have had these experiences come back with a purpose for their life that often takes them in a new direction.

Some of us have to be figuratively "hit over the head," that is, to come uncomfortably close to death, before we see the light. However, I don't advise the reader to try this at home—to venture too close to that slippery edge between this life and some other dimension—because the laws of the universe include a measure of uncertainty in the equations; and there is no guarantee that a person would be able to come back and complete the unique set of lessons offered by the world as it exists today in this lifetime.

"I don't want to die here." The compelling word for me in that second thought was "here." What did that mean? As in our dreams, where the subconscious mind communicates to us through symbols, maybe the word "here" was a symbol of a bigger part of my life. Did it mean, here in Boston, for an exiled lover of the American West? Did it mean here as a graduate student on track to be a scientist and academic researcher? Or here in my current undeveloped state of being? As it turned out, it was all of the above.

In terms of the enneagram of healing, that was for me a profound point-three experience on that snowy morning forty years ago. And if it wasn't for the heavy snowstorm that the universe provided, I probably wouldn't have exerted myself to the point of passing out, and in that hypothetical case might not have received the shock that resulted, which changed the direction of my life. I don't believe this is an example of determinism in the philosophical sense; it was more like the fortuitous confluence of two intersecting processes, one internal and one external. A "mechano-coinciding" event, the sense of which Gurdjieff so aptly embodied in that phrase.

The other strong impression of my point-three experience was the awakening in the police car. It was clear in that moment that my survival depended upon those two people, the policeman and my wife, offering their most focused attention on my behalf. Without their efforts, there is no way that I would have survived that day. This continues to be a source of deep gratitude for me, especially since I recently became aware that averaged over the last forty years, about 4,000 people per year have died of acute asthmatic episodes in America. In other words, over 160,000 people have died in a similar way since January 1, 1971.

Gazing a little further into point-three we can see from the story recounted above that there is hazard at this step of the healing octave. When people wait too long to decide that they need help, then even with the best support of the outside world they sometime don't make it in time to receive the hands-on assistance that would have come at point-four. Or they may survive the trip to the hospital, but not live long enough to recover from the heroic intervention that happens in the ER, especially for victims of heart attacks, strokes, aneurysms, and severe asthma attacks.

There are specific efforts that help one to navigate the Mi-Fa interval and arrive intact at point-four, just as there were other efforts for 0→1 and 1→2. At the Mi-Fa interval one needs faith that the right decision was made, trust that the world will provide what is needed to actualize the decision, and hope that it will eventually lead to the result one visualized along the 2→8 inner line.

Faith, trust, and hope help bring the person through the shock at point-three. Then one may experience gratitude and openness to receiving help as they approach point-four.

The enemies here are the opposites of the above named impulses: doubt, lack of trust, and dread—all of which lead to increased tension and anxiety. These latter are the last things a person needs at this stage. Relaxation and letting go of anxiety are the antidotes that are appropriate for those internal obstacles at this stage, and actually at every step in the process. Relaxation not only has multiple physiological benefits in a crisis, but it releases the mind to access or receive information that could be crucial.

Occasionally when a certain type of new patient arrives at my office, which is in effect arriving at point-four, I can sometimes sense suspicion and mistrust in their field, which heightens the fear and apprehension that they were already feeling. My task in those situations is to relax myself, as fully as I can, and not be infected by their tension. When my inner relaxation and sense of presence reach a certain threshold, I often notice these types of patients begin to relax and let go a little.

However, as I have observed repeatedly, the ability of patients to deeply relax is a learned skill, which requires specific directed efforts and much serious practice over many years. Chronically tense people often say, "I can't relax," and they are right, because they have never worked at the technique. But it can be learned for those willing to work at it.

Another asthmatic crisis I went through has relevance here. This was the last, that is, the most recent scary attack that I have endured, and it occurred on a chilly winter night in 1983:

I was sitting on the floor next to the wood stove in our house near Aurora, Oregon late in the evening after the rest of my family was asleep. I don't remember the circumstances that led to the severity of my symptoms that night; I just remember my condition getting worse and worse to the point where I was gasping and had no breath even to call for help. I was on my own, but fortunately I had taken some prednisone, and was hoping it would take effect before too long. Even more fortunately, I had by this time learned the techniques of Work on oneself. As I sat there gasping, I relaxed myself as much as I could, especially my mind. I noticed that even a single anxious thought was enough to intensify the gasping and the lung spasms almost to the point where I could again feel the strange effects of oxygen deprivation. I had no choice but to completely quiet my mind, relax the parts of my body not being used and simply wait for my breathing to regain its equilibrium. By then I knew first-hand what would happen if I gave in to panic in that situation.

I not only prayed for help that night but as the gasping finally subsided a little, I made a promise to my body that if it would just allow me a few more years living in that damp and moldy place where it was so difficult for me to breathe, until something could be crystallized in terms of my personal evolution and study at Two Rivers Farm, then I would move to a place where it would be more possible for me to thrive, and where I could actualize what I was learning.

Then little by little my bronchial tubes opened up, and I was given another reprieve. This time it was the Work efforts I had made during the previous ten years that contributed to saving my life.

The reason that I recounted this experience here, is primarily to give an example of how essential work at relaxation can be, not only for healing at point-four but even for survival itself.

Soon after the night described above, where I again came too close to the edge, I made a therapeutic discovery. After reading an article in a medical journal, I realized it was the synthetic broncho-dilating drugs which I had relied upon so heavily for the previous twelve years, that had caused the asthmatic spasms to have become so severe. Once I stopped taking those pills—totally and forever—never again was there an attack of that order of frightening severity.

So I was able to survive in the Willamette Valley for several more years, dividing my energies between my Work activities with the group, my chiropractic practice, my life at home with my wife and two children, and an occasional respite for my lungs on periodic trips to the desert. In fact, it was almost exactly nine years later, a complete cycle of the enneagram, that my family and I moved over the mountains to the high, dry plateau of Central Oregon.

CHAPTER 3

# Point Four

Point-four, the note Fa of the octave, is interesting in the healing process for many reasons. For one, it represents the beginning of treatment, the initial contact with the doctor or therapy. In a sense, the whole right side of the enneagram circle, from point-one onward, is a preparation for the treatment that is initiated at this step in the process.

The key effort for the patient at point-four is one of submission. In order to bridge the gap and arrive safely at point-five, that is, to bring about a tangible improvement in their condition, the patient needs to submit for a time to the will of the doctor. And this can only happen when there is a relationship of trust, or at least openness, established between the doctor and patient.

In the event that the patient were to have resistance to the doctor and his/her methods, there would be little chance for a positive outcome. When patients reject key parts of the doctor's recommendations, for example, they are willing to take this remedy or supplement but not the other ones, then the patient is, as we say, suffering from the "help me, don't help me" syndrome. The psychology of this particular ambivalence may have something to do with the fear of letting go of control, or the effects of past traumatic experiences with doctors in general.

It is true that there will be more benefit if a patient participates in the planning and execution of the treatment, instead of being totally passive and allowing the doctor to do whatever. The patient's main task at point-four is to be reasonably certain that they can trust the doctor, and then allow themselves to relax and let go.

Sometimes an openness to the doctor, and his/her treatment protocol, is facilitated by the workings of the 4→2 inner line (see Figure 4-1 on page 54). At point-four the patient can reconnect with the decision made at point-two. There can be a reaffirmation of the intention, and an instantaneous connection with the reason why the choice was made to see that particular doctor or healer. Often the choice is made because of a referral from a friend or relative who received help from the chosen doctor. However, occasionally the patient—beginning to traverse the 4→5 interval, and having an attack of doubts or second thoughts after the initial contact with the doctor—can be reassured by remembering the enthusiasm of the person who referred them. In fact, over the years I have seen a number of easily discouraged patients who continued with treatment after the initial visit or two only because of persuasive verbal reassurance by their referring friend or relative.

There are many variations in patients' reactions at point-four. Occasionally, the patient will really have made a bad choice and it soon becomes clear that they aren't going to be helped by that doctor. The only option for them in that case is to "bite-the-bullet" and literally go back to point-two and make a different choice.

However, without a measure of discernment, patients tend to repeat their mistakes. Many, unfortunately become stuck in that cycle of 2→4→2→4→2...., rejecting one doctor after another, searching in vain for someone who can help a very difficult or intractable problem. The mantra for this subset of patients is, "I've tried everything." In reality they might have tried a few types of treatment, but haven't yet found a healing system that works for them. But enduring the cycle of 2→4→2... can be very discouraging and exhausting and often patients lose heart before they ever find any real help. In this case, they learn to exist with their debilitating condition because of its familiarity and the routines they have established around it, so that their suffering becomes the path of least resistance. Then their motto is, "I'm just going to have to live with it."

Whenever I hear these phrases from a new acquaintance or a new patient, and the attitude that underlies them, I try to inspire them to keep searching. Defeat can only happen when one gives up. As long as they keep trying and are determined enough in their intention, sooner or later what they need will present itself. I have seen this happen many times.

I sometimes ask these people, "what's the worst that can happen? Death? But we're all going to die anyway, so you might as well die struggling to find what you need, than be resigned to a life of suffering." Healing does occur when one finally encounters what they need.

In the mid-1980's I studied briefly with the Tibetan Buddhist physician, Chakdud Tulku Rinpoche, who used to tell his students, "disease is like a monster or an entity that is clinging to you and living on your energy. It's important that you continue to battle the monster and defeat it before you die, otherwise you will probably have to face the same monster again in the next lifetime." If one takes this advice to heart, it can be a great source of motivation, no matter what the "monster" is.

When I have been able to help patients who have become discouraged and jaded from previous medical failures, it is always heartwarming to watch their emotional state change from the initial skepticism, to a grudging willingness to agree to a treatment plan, to amazement and wonder, to an ebullient gratitude, and finally they sing my praises to their friends and family, greatly exaggerating the help they received.

Another scenario that occurs all too often at point-four, because of our peculiar medical system, is when a patient only resorts to the services of a particular doctor, usually an M.D., in order to refill a prescription, for example, for pain pills, migraine medication, hormones, anti-depressants, or one of many other drugs upon which the patient has become dependent. In many of these cases there is no real relationship of trust with the doctor; instead there is a kind of co-dependency where the two people are using each other for their own interests. The latter is a situation where it is improbable that the patient's octave of healing will proceed much further than point-five, and if it did, it would be in spite of the dysfunction in the relationship established at point-four. In fact, anytime a patient has the attitude that they are enduring or tolerating a doctor for an ulterior motive, or because they are afraid to make a change even though they are not receiving real help, this is an obvious red flag that their octave is in serious danger of being stalled before it reaches point-seven. In other words they may never even reach a symptom-free status.

The chances of completing the healing octave increase dramatically when point-four, Fa, is sounded on a strong and vibrant note. And this means, in light of the above, a good feeling and an open heart toward the doctor or therapy that is chosen by the patient.

A doctor or therapist may be an expert in their field, widely recognized for their publications or the teaching of their technique, esteemed by their peers, etc., but if doctors who have achieved this kind of success turn out to be too busy to take the extra time to establish a kindred relationship with an especially needy patient, this may be another indication of trouble. On the other hand, it is true that doctors in this elite category are creative and innovative and will bring some patients to point-five in a more direct and certain way.

However, in my experience it is advisable for a patient to find a more humble, but competent practitioner who is capable of taking the extra time to make that essential emotional connection with their patients. Then healing can happen on multiple levels, with an increased probability of continuing beyond point-five, as we shall see. Also, the doctor who takes the time to probe into the early details of an illness or injury—details that might have been overlooked by a busier practitioner, and that the patients themselves may not remember upon the initial inquiry—this doctor may discover important clues that could lead to a breakthrough for the patient's healing.

Whenever I see patients for whom the "good feeling" mentioned above—that intangible something that draws people to each other and creates a kind of empathy—is mutually present, this quality of relationship in itself evokes the confidence in me that the patient will receive help, not only with the acute problems from which they currently suffer, but with almost any malady that might happen to them later. These future imbalances can most often be nipped-in-the-bud, not only because they are detected at the earliest stages, but because there is that connection between the patient and me that transcends conventional understanding.

I call these special people my "spirit patients," because of that mysterious bond we share that opens up new energetic possibilities. This type of patient is rare, but when I'm fortunate enough to treat one, its as though I ascend into that proverbial "zone" when I'm working on them— totally focused, inwardly quiet, and certain that they are receiving exactly what they need at that moment. This is possible because of an enhanced openness and trust between us, that relaxes some unconscious constriction present in either or both of us that would otherwise impede the healing process.

On this topic of "enhanced openness," I wish to relate a story of a "point-four experience" on the enneagram of spiritual development, that was told to me concerning the first meeting of a student with her spiritual teacher. Point-four on the octave of inner Work is analogous to point-four on the octave of healing; the first contact with the doctor is very similar to the first contact with one's mentor. (See Figure Ap-2 on page 119.)

The circumstances pertaining to how I learned about this point-four experience are really part of the story, so I will include those as well:

In early 1978 I was part of a large group of students from Two Rivers Farm who drove from Oregon down to the San Francisco Bay Area one weekend to see the West Coast premiere of the film, *Meetings With Remarkable Men*. The movie was the brainchild of Jeanne de Salzmann, who was also in attendance, having traveled all the way from Paris for the showing. After the movie was over, there was a reception in a large room in the grand old theater. Madam de Salzmann noticed a group of about ten of us from Oregon standing together and told her companions, elders from New York and San Francisco, "I want to speak to the 'young people'." So she walked over to us and was immediately surrounded by our little group, and proceeded to listen to our reactions to the film and answer our questions in turn. It was an unexpected, once-in-a-lifetime opportunity.

The comment that I conveyed to her was the result of a strong impression I had during a scene where the young Gurdjieff realized that he needed to travel to a certain country to find a long-lost monastery. I remember the feeling that came over me, watching that scene, when his friend said something like, "you can't go there, a civil war is going on in that country." After which, Gurdjieff, with a penetrating look off into the distance, simply replied, "I must go."

What I felt after I heard those words was a fear that passed through me, when I undeniably cognized how serious one's search for truth needs to be, serious enough to face death, if that's what it takes.

So I told Mme. de Salzmann that I experienced a very real fear during that scene when I questioned whether my own commitment could be that total.

She just smiled and said, "Why be afraid?"

For a moment or two we looked into each other's eyes. She was 89 years old at the time and her eyes weren't exactly clear the way a child's eyes are, yet they weren't really cloudy either. I had never seen eyes like that; it was like looking into a deep lake.

Then she spoke again and said, "When I first met Mr. Gurdjieff we looked into each other's eyes and I'll never forget that moment if I live to be 200 years old. I knew I was *home*," (she emphasized the word *home*) "There would never again be anything to fear."

She may have spoken a little more, but by that point I was already filled to capacity, not just from her words and what they meant, but from her energy as well, and I couldn't contain any more. The next thing I remember, she was speaking to another man in our group, a big man who was about 6' 1" and weighed about 230 pounds, and who started sobbing like a child in the intensity of his emotion, standing in front of Mme. de Salzmann. At that point I left the knot of people around her so I could digest my own experience and so the person who was behind me would have a chance to ask her question.

I have pondered that brief exchange several times over the years and have found new meaning more than once, but for this discussion the relevant aspect is the total or "enhanced" openness she immediately felt in the presence of Gurdjieff, along with a conviction, an intuitive certainty, that he would provide her all she needed.

The quality of that first encounter with her teacher produced such a resounding note that she accompanied him for the next thirty years until his death, and then devoted the remaining 52 years of her life to carrying on his Work, completing her own octave, and in the process being a wisdom-holder and an inspiration for thousands of seekers in many parts of the world.

That first meeting between Mme de. Salzmann and Gurdjieff was truly one of the most extraordinary "point-four experiences" of the last hundred years. Others that come to mind were the meeting of Carlos

Casteneda with the Yaqui shaman, Don Juan; and the meeting of Tom Brown with his Apache master, Stalking Wolf.

The word, doctor, as many readers may be aware, means teacher. It comes from the Latin root, *docere*, which means, to teach. A strong point-four experience between a seeker and his/her spiritual teacher, as I noted earlier, has much in common with a patient's first encounter with his/her doctor. The patient, after this experience, may not only be helped with their physical dysfunction, but can learn many things from the doctor. And in those instances where there is a strong enough experience, and if it is the right time in the patient's life, they may wish to emulate the doctor, and even "walk in his footsteps," as it were.

This latter phenomenon actually happened to me in 1975 when I began treatment with a chiropractor/naturopath/acupuncturist in Boulder, Colorado, named Tim Binder. This was my first foray into the world of Alternative Health Care, and it affected me in many ways. Not only did my asthmatic condition dramatically and rapidly improve, which stunned me at the time, but I was deeply moved by the overall approach: the stimulation of my body's own resources by needles inserted in special points which produced some mysterious energetic change; the chiropractic adjustments that released blockages in my nervous system; and the botanical and homeopathic remedies that acted on my internal chemistry in a specific yet gentle way—all these methods were consistent with my life-long instinctive tendency to trust nature whenever possible. They also provided a long overdue and effective alternative to my previous habit of relying upon prescription medications—or "poison drugs," as the Chinese traditionally called them—to relax my bronchial tubes. And these natural methods provided an alternative to my other habit of waiting until there was a crisis and then rushing to the emergency room. One more decisive benefit of this kind of natural treatment was that it opened a door about which I had not known. It represented a 180° change of direction for me to look inside myself with the new concept that what I eat, how I hold myself in a postural sense, what influences I subject myself to, and even how I react emotionally, all affect my health—more than I ever imagined—and that these choices are my responsibility.

Except for occasional acute and severe asthmatic episodes at that time, I was an otherwise active and healthy 30 year-old, unaware that any special kind of vigilance in relation to the maintenance of my body was necessary. To me the asthma was an anomaly that I believed would eventually disappear on its own. So until my treatments from Dr. Binder, I ignored this anomaly during my intermittent healthy periods, and forgot or denied that there was a significant problem.

No medical doctor had ever questioned my diet or life-style except for obvious habits, like smoking cigarettes. I was struck that this alternative doctor was concerned about details and subtleties that no other health professional in my experience had ever noticed; and the whole way he approached my care was unprecedented.

After a few treatments, he could see that I had both the talent and the interest to be an alternative doctor like himself. He was the one who suggested that I enroll in chiropractic college, but it took me well over a year to actually make the decision.

Unlike Mme. de Salzmann's meeting with Mr. Gurdjieff, my point-four experience with Dr. Binder was not immediately life-changing. The inner change of direction was a gradual process that entailed overcoming much resistance over a long period of time.

In fact, everyone's experience at point-four will be different; there are a spectrum of possibilities. What they all have in common is simply the arrival at that gravity-center marker in the overall process; the beginning of a relationship with someone whose purpose is to restore one's health, or to facilitate the transformation of one's being, if it is spiritual help one is seeking.

As such, point-four is another deflection, and going beyond it marks another change in direction of one's effort (as do all the points). Before this, one's energy was directed toward placing oneself into the position of receiving help (point-two→point-four, or the Mi–Fa interval); after one has arrived there, the new direction, the 4→5 interval, has an entirely different character, again with different kinds of efforts required.

Chapter 4

# The 4→5 Interval

In the oft-quoted enneagram of the "The Kitchen as a Cosmos," from John Bennett's book, *Enneagram Studies*[1], the 4→5 interval occurs when "the bread is in the oven." It is the period of time when the cooks do not have direct control over their materials. They set the conditions, then have to let go and allow the fire to act on the dough in its own way.

Likewise for the healing octave, patients have done what they can to transfer themselves into the care of a doctor or healer, now they have to let go and allow the treatment to work. The effort here, as I mentioned earlier, is one of submission.

In the octave of spiritual development, a similar effort is needed on the part of the seeker at this point when he/she begins work in a group. For a certain number of years, at least until the teaching is absorbed, the disciple must submit his/her self-will to the teacher's will, or in other words be completely obedient to the teacher's suggestions. This concept is obvious to those who have lived in a monastery or Worked in a "school," but to a secular-type, it would probably raise their hackles. One reason for submission is that in order to develop real will, or obey a higher will when one can be in touch with it, one must first have the ability to control the impulsive and unruly self-will. It is next to impossible to do this by oneself without help from a teacher or guide. As with the doctor-patient

---
1  John G. Bennett, *Enneagram Studies*, Weiser, 1983, p. 25.

relationship, the seeker must have sufficient trust and openness to make these efforts.

But in both cases, discernment—both instinctive and rational—must be in readiness, "waiting in the wings" so to speak. As a process proceeds along the 4→5 interval, the bread may begin to burn, the spiritual teacher may turn out to have some irreconcilable weakness that would make it psychologically destructive for the student to continue, or the doctor's treatment for one reason or another may not be working, although this latter case needs further clarification.

There is a phenomenon that often occurs at this initial stage of treatment, known in alternative health jargon as a "healing crisis," or sometimes experienced simply as "it gets worse before it gets better." This can happen when there is a dysfunction of the internal organs, often related to a toxic burden in the body. "Toxins" can be heavy metals, which are grossly overabundant in our air, food, water, and materials in this age; they can be poisonous organic chemicals, also grossly overabundant and grossly under-detected in modern times; toxins can be waste materials from bacterial, viral, or parasitic infections, or wastes from the patient's own metabolism if the organs of elimination are failing in any way. The human body, faced with a continual toxic overload, attempts to sequester or hide these poisons by storing them in certain cells where they will do minimal harm. After the initial treatment, when the organs of elimination begin to function at an increased level, the body's internal controller begins to dump these stored toxins into the circulation hoping to be finally rid of them.

Unfortunately, there is often an internal miscalculation or a temporary return of the original dysfunction, and the circulating toxins, unable to be totally eliminated, can produce all sorts of symptoms, occasionally making the patient feel worse than when they started treatment, for a short time. If the patient isn't educated or forewarned of this possibility, they can become discouraged, assume the treatment is not working, and discontinue what would have really helped them had they persevered. Unfortunately, mainstream medicine at present is largely unaware of the concept of the healing crisis, and offers no help with understanding or dealing with this problem in terms of ancillary detoxification methods.

One ramification of the above discussion for the 4→5 interval is the issue of discouragement when the patient doesn't see immediate results. If the patient has never experienced a healing crisis, they have no data to discriminate between that phenomenon and a real worsening of the condition. Here again is a place for intuition, asking for guidance, and for trust and submission to the doctor, if it feels right.

To traverse this region of the octave, ultimately one needs to persist until a tangible result is achieved. Sometimes one can be fortunate, and the result will be quick, but usually it is a gradual process, and then persistence is the best ally.

This lowest segment of the circle, the 4→5 interval, the bridge between the right side and the left side of the enneagram circle, is in a way the crux of the whole healing process. Other words with this "cru" root are equally descriptive of the transition, as crucible or crucial. (See Figure 4-1 on page 54, for this part of the enneagram.)

There is a whole spectrum of possible scenarios of the action of this interval which we will continue to discuss.

But first, on the topic of submission, there is one more aspect to mention, and this is the extreme example of agreeing to a major surgery. On the operating table, one's life for a time is in the hands of a surgeon(s) and their team and any discernment in this case must come beforehand. Once on the table there is no going back, no opting out, at least in terms of the patient's discretion. One wakes up and perhaps arrives at point-five with the obstruction unblocked, the malignancy removed, the former pain lessened, the shattered bone pieced together, or whatever. But all too often the surgery doesn't relieve the problem, again for many reasons. Perhaps it was ill-advised to begin with, maybe the surgeon or assistant made a tragic mistake, perhaps the problem turned out to be too complex to repair, or for some other unforeseen and unknown reason the patient awakened still in that limbo between point-four and point-five.

By the way, I must add here that part of my aim in writing this monograph has been to be as non-judgmental as I can in terms of the advocacy of one form of healing over another; in another words I am attempting to put my own biases aside, which of course is not so easy. The different types of treatments available in my lifetime are described only to provide examples of the successive stages of the octave. And of course I have more data about some than others. But surgery is a great example of the 4→5 transformation because of the forced submission and the complete abdication of control and self-will on the part of the patient, analogous to the bread going into the oven in the kitchen enneagram.

But if I may make an exception to my rule, I will voice a concern about surgery in general that bothers me, and that is, in terms of the healing transformative process, surgery requires a total passivity on the part of the patient. Obviously, there are times when there is no viable alternative to a surgical procedure in order to save someone's life in an emergency. We are fortunate to have this option available; and emergency surgery is a real achievement of twentieth century civilization. But in general, if a patient can participate in the process starting from point-four, it is a help, because each subsequent stage from this point requires more and more inner activity and self-discipline. And as one goes beyond point-seven and especially point-eight, there are less and less ways a doctor or another person can intervene in order to help the process continue. In other words, if one's aim is to complete the octave, one needs to be active and participate at least by point-five.

An example of the need to be active, as early in the process as possible, comes from the so called lap-band surgery for extremely obese people. In this procedure, a band is placed around the upper part of the stomach to shrink its size and thus prevent too much food from entering at each meal. Some patients lose scores of pounds after this surgery, but others, including one that I know, couldn't lose more than 20-30 pounds—out of 90-100 that she needed to lose—in over a year, because she couldn't muster the discipline to refrain from eating junk foods and eating as much as her shrunken stomach would hold.

In terms of the enneagram, if one is stuck psychologically at point-four, being unable to control their habitual impulses, and are passively carried across the bridge to point-five, they would still need to face the same obstacles going from 5→6→7, only then there are new difficulties, as we shall see later.

Another example of the passivity issue is with heroin addicts who are given methadone as a way of replacing one bad habit with another one only slightly less addictive and dangerous; or cigarette smokers opting to chew nicotine gum or wear patches in attempt to quit their habit.

My purpose in listing these examples is not necessarily to advocate one form of treatment over another, rather to point out how excessive passivity at the 4→5 interval may be counterproductive in the long run, that is, if one has an aim to return to optimum health. It's as though, in the above examples, allegorically one is carried over to the promised land but has brought all their old baggage with them.

On the other hand, the more I ponder this question of passivity at the 4→5 interval, the more I see that it is not so "black and white," because some passivity is necessary at this stage. This is the step where one submits to a treatment. In general terms, something is done to me, and I relax and allow it to happen.

Being too active at this interval is also ill-advised in most cases. For example people try to cure themselves of musculo-skeletal injuries with exercises, and in my long experience, this doesn't work the majority of the time. Exercising an injured muscle or ligament usually makes it worse, just as trying to put weight on a broken bone before the new bone material is stable would undermine the chances of proper healing. Advancing from 4→5 is a time for some passivity and a time to allow the chosen method to work on one's organism. A time to work at being, instead of doing. It is question of finding a balance between active and passive participation.

In some cases, as with infectious diseases that can be self-limiting, one is simply compelled to go to bed and allow the healing that is taking place from within to happen. All one needs to do in this case is feed the immune system the specific nutrients it needs for maximal function and put one's mind and body to rest.

The mind, and particularly negative imagination, anxiety, worry, etc. can be huge impediments at every step, but especially this one. These energy drains act like brakes on the healing engine. Taking one's mind off the problem during the initial treatment allows the internal energy to flow where it is needed.

Dr. Edward Bach, who developed the Flower Remedies in England in the 1930's, believed that disease actually resulted from a conflict between, as he put it, the soul and the personality. He developed a series of 38 different flower extracts designed to treat the emotional imbalances that in his philosophy were the underlying cause of physical ailments. The vibrations, or electromagnetic pattern of an individual flower in a homeopathic sense are thought to act on a specific emotional problem, such as fear, indecision, worry, jealousy, etc. In the words of his biographer, Nora Weeks,

> "When he treated the personalities and feelings of his patients, their unhappiness and physical distress would be alleviated, and the natural healing potential in their bodies was unblocked and allowed to work once more."[2]

There is no overestimating the tremendous power of healing inherent in the human body, once the mind, with its almost constant siphoning and wasting of energy, is to put to rest. In fact this latter idea has a foundation in physiology, which involves the opposing balance of the sympathetic and parasympathetic parts of the autonomic nervous system. The sympathetic side is dominant during activity and stress, and causes the secretion of two adrenal hormones, cortisol and adrenalin. These hormones mediate the famous "fight or flight" response, that originally were reactions to mortal danger in a biological sense. However, in today's accelerated, "stressed-out" conditions of life, the adrenal hormones are chronically elevated in many people, occasionally to the point where the adrenal glands themselves become exhausted. Also, the sympathetic nervous system causes blood vessels to become constricted, and the breathing and heart rate to become accelerated. Some fraction of blood is shunted away from the organs and into the large muscle groups. Healing, during stressful events, is put on hold.

In contrast, the parasympathetic nervous system is the active force in the opposite circumstances, that is during periods of relaxation, resting, during and after a meal (parasympathetic nerves turn on digestion), and anytime one is outwardly passive and quiet, especially during meditation. When the parasympathetic nervous system is dominant, healing is facilitated. On the opposite extreme, when there are frequent stressful thought patterns and emotional reactions that simulate real violence, panic, or shock to some degree there will be corresponding sympathetic dominance that severely impedes healing.

---

2 Weeks, Nora, *The Medical Discoveries of Edward Bach, Physician.*

To reiterate, the power of the mind at the 4→5 interval is the power to relax, disengage, and allow the acute problem to be resolved by the magnificent healing ability of the body, augmented by whatever external help is available. This is probably the most powerful way a patient can participate and be active in the process at this step.

In my own repeating cycle of acute asthmatic episodes in the 1970's, I learned this principle quite by accident. In late 1974 my wife and I had just spent several trying, or as it is said now "challenging" days with my parents in Los Angeles, and afterward drove up to the San Francisco Bay Area to visit some old friends. I was already extremely asthmatic when we left Los Angeles, but by the time we arrived in Oakland, I could barely breathe, and my broncho-dilating drugs weren't working. I urgently needed to go to a hospital. But remember, this was 25 years before the advent of cell phones, GPS devices, etc. Driving on the freeway, we had to rely on paper maps and memory, and all we could remember at that time was that there was a Kaiser-Permanente hospital somewhere near downtown Oakland, that was easy to access from the freeway. We weren't sure that they would accept me as a patient since I was not a member, but we took a chance, found the hospital and as it turned out they did take me in and brought me to a bed in a module in the emergency room. After a cursory exam, I was given a shot of adrenalin, then pretty much left there on my own. Because of my earlier experiences at the great teaching hospitals in Boston three years earlier, it became clear rather quickly that this facility was way behind the times, and that relative to my dire needs, they really didn't know what they were doing. Doctors in the 1950's used to give me adrenalin shots, and they had stopped being effective in my case long ago.

I remember the moment that I realized this—that I wasn't going to get any help there unless I was able to direct my own care, which was woefully unlikely. I couldn't even get a nurse's attention. Suddenly, it all became kind of overwhelming. I felt a wave of fatigue overtake me and I just stopped fighting it. I lied down on my side and just kind of gave up and dozed off. Within a minute, a huge plug of thick mucus came out of my throat. There was no coughing or hacking; it just spontaneously released. Two minutes later, another one even larger came out and I sat up a little surprised and puzzled, but realized that my breathing was returning to normal and I was going to be alright. It wasn't difficult to conclude that when I completely relaxed and my anxious mind turned itself off momentarily, that the initial stage of healing just happened.

However, it would roughly be another nine years (the 1983 experience that I mentioned in the previous chapter) before I was able to intentionally relax, that is, more or less consciously practice the technique of deep relaxation, instead of depending on accidental circumstances.

In summary, going through this interval and arriving at point-five represents emerging from the acute or severe part of the illness or injury to a freer place where there has been some tangible improvement. The direction of the journey will change again and one will embark on the path to restoring their health in a more complete way.

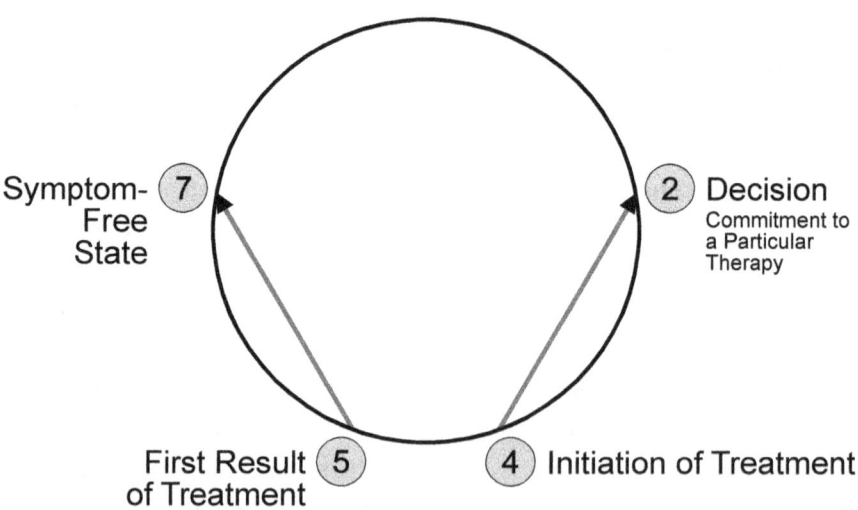

**Figure 4-1,** *Partial Enneagram focusing on the 4→5 Interval and associated Inner Lines*

The 4→5 interval (the fourth stopinder) is where the treatment—one or many—is actually taking place, and the interval is crossed when the patient begins to perceive a positive change in his/her condition. The 4→2 inner line represents a revisiting or a reconsideration of the decision to choose this therapy; and the 5→7 inner line allows one, after they have achieved the initial result, to anticipate and imagine that they can really be free of their pain, or other symptoms, if they continue with their healing. Unfortunately, the 5→7 inner line can also enable one to have the illusion that they have already reached point-seven before making any real effort to do so, as we will discuss in the next chapter.

## Chapter 5
# Point Five and the 5→7 Interval

Passing from the right side of the enneagram circle around the bottom to the left side (4→5) is a significant transition, and I hope the reader now has a sense of that. But before discussing point-five in detail, there is one more aspect to the approach to point-five that I will mention first.

There is a certain moment just beyond the bottom of the circle on the way to point-five where one begins to feel that the treatment is working, that relief is on the way, that one is "over the hump." The latter is a relatively accurate metaphor, because leaving point-four can be like struggling up a hill. Then there is a discreet moment in this step of the process where the hill has been crested and the feeling of relief begins to be felt.

It is like that point in a sporting event or game when one suddenly knows with certainty which team (or individual) is going to win. This moment may come earlier or later or occasionally not until the end, but it is a definite landmark and a turning point in one's relationship to the situation.

In other words, at the approach to point-five there is some definite, observable improvement or relief, an initial result of the treatment of the acute problem.

Point-five in the musical octave is the note Sol, which vibrationally is about halfway between the lower and higher Do. In a literal sense one might expect the halfway point to be the space between the fourth and fifth note. But in the musical octave it comes at the fifth note. The chord Do-Sol is called a "fifth" and is half an octave. I don't fully understand the significance of this phenomenon except that it has to do with the asymmetry of the Mi-Fa and the Si-Do intervals.

Likewise in the healing enneagram, as the patient approaches point-five, and has had the experience that something has definitely changed, that there has been a real improvement—at this stage they actually are only halfway to "wholeness." In a subtle but objective sense, a new kind of work starts at this point.

The point-five experience is essentially the feeling of the change in one's condition. The confirming verbalization that I sometimes hear from patients after this initial period, is simply "It feels different."

I sometimes respond, "That's a good sign, it means we have begun a sequence of healing."

Occasionally, a long-standing pain will be gone, sometimes just lessened in intensity. In some cases, the pain will not only subside to some degree, but move to a different part of the body. In both cases a blockage will have been cleared and energy will begin to flow again. Sometimes there may be secondary or even tertiary blockages or consequences of the main problem, and the patient might not feel a dramatic change, nor a very noticeable improvement, until the second or third level of obstruction is cleared.

By analogy, the above variation is similar on another scale to the after-effects of a multiple vehicle collision on a busy highway, where for example, several cars or trucks have completely blocked the road and traffic is backed up for miles. Eventually the tow-trucks and highway police are able to clear one lane for traffic to pass through. The first cars in line will start moving, but others waiting over a mile back from the incident may not notice the change for several minutes or perhaps until a second lane is cleared.

In like manner after being treated either by a chiropractor, acupuncturist, energy healer, or other physical medicine specialist who works directly on the body, there may be a real change for a patient even after a few minutes of the first treatment. But there still may be an energy bottleneck, as is the case after the crash on the highway. In both cases however, something will begin to flow again, and sooner or later the patient will perceive the change.

The cognition that some improvement has happened usually triggers an emotional response as well. In fact all three "brains" of the patient participate in the arrival at point-five.

As an example of a point-five experience, I will site a most unusual experience that happened to Lance Armstrong on one of his Tour de France races, that was related to me in a class taught by his chiropractor, Dr. Jeff Spencer. (Keep in mind that this particular story is from the doctor's point of view):

Lance had a bad fall during one leg of the race one year and injured his hip. By evening it had tightened up so much that he literally could not walk. But he needed to appear at some kind of awards dinner in less than twenty minutes. So he summoned his chiropractor to his trailer and told him the situation. Dr. Spencer proceeded to give Lance a brief exam and a quick but thorough treatment according to his standard protocol. There was no noticeable change after the treatment, and now they only had about 7 or 8 minutes left. Lance still could barely put weight on the affected side. So Dr. Spencer unleashed his creativity and tried another technique based upon his evaluation of the injury, and then another. Still there was no viable result, and now they were down to 2-3 minutes before needing to leave the trailer in order to arrive at the dinner on time. Keep in mind that both of these people were ultra-competitive, highly successful and super-competent with their skills, and failure was not a part of their mindset. It was totally unacceptable. But time was running out, and Dr. Spencer confessed to us that this is when he began to pray, which he normally reserved only for dire situations. With about one minute left, Dr. Spencer's ordinary mind gave up, shut down, and his instincts took over; or maybe it was his subconscious mind, or maybe something else, but he just grabbed Lance's leg and with a particular lift and rotation he yanked as hard as he could on the leg to adjust the hip the old-fashioned way. He heard a crack so loud, his first thought was that he had caused a fracture. Holding his breath, in a figurative sense, he told Lance to stand on it and take a step or two. When Lance complied in a very tentative way, Dr. Spencer asked him how it felt, and Lance replied, "I don't know."

That is the last thing a chiropractor wants to hear in a situation like that because if a patient can't sense a positive change, it usually means either there isn't one, or now it is worse, and the patient is reluctant to admit it. (I have "been there and done that" myself although not ever in such a dramatic way).

Lance continued gingerly taking little steps around the trailer and after a minute or so was aware that his hip joint had been repositioned and restored almost to normal, and it was beginning to feel better with every step. Dr. Spencer let out a deep sigh, and together they walked to the dining area only a minute or two late for the presentation.

There are many things to be learned from this story, and many tangents onto which I am tempted to wander, but I will limit myself to one, and that is how interesting it is that there are hundreds millions of people who are aware that Lance Armstrong and the American Postal Team won the Tour de France seven times (and of course now aware of the doping issues also), but almost no one by comparison is aware of the heroics of healing that went on behind the scenes to keep those cyclists racing, not only the one time cited above but many, many times for almost all the team members throughout all those years.

Another aspect is that one can see how a person in super physical condition and hyper-motivated to regain his optimal functioning, can traverse the enneagram circle from point-one to point-five in a few hours and on to point-seven by the following morning.

Based upon what I learned from Dr. Spencer, Lance probably slept that night with a special blanket grounded electrically to the Earth, to speed up the healing process (this was one of many avant-garde or experimental procedures that Dr. Spencer embraced in order to achieve that "edge" over the competition) so that by the time of the next part of the race, Lance was close to being at point-seven, where he was able to function normally, but by no means completely healed.

Looking ahead, point-seven is experienced as that stage where one is asymptomatic and can once again function almost normally, but is still very vulnerable to re-injury or relapse.

The above story is an example of what is possible in an extreme case, when two extraordinary people working together completely focus their whole being on the desired outcome. But it is after all, near one end of the spectrum of possible outcomes and in most cases it takes much longer to ascend beyond point-five.

Another way chiropractic patients have of expressing their point-five experience, is the utterance, "Now my back doesn't hurt until I try to do something."

In my own case when I am at point-five I can breathe normally as long as I am sitting still but as soon as I expend any energy or walk too fast the wheezing returns.

The usual scenario is that at point-five there has been noticeable improvement and relief but the person can't yet function normally, thus there are still confounding issues to be considered.

## The 5→7 interval

The journey from point-five through point-six to point-seven (the Sol-La interval) is one of the most interesting and complex steps of the whole process. The complexity is a result of several factors:

1) On the left side of the enneagram, that is, in the second half of the process, the energies are finer and the transformations, although definite, are more difficult to identify and characterize. This is like the difference between, for example, powder snow and a wetter snow, which is an obvious distinction for a skier but to a person growing up in a tropical climate, they are both just snow. Likewise, for a person previously healthy all their life up to a present crisis, the distinctions in their experience between their first improvement (point-five), a return to feeling no symptoms at all(point-seven), and a more stable and robust level of health (point-eight ), may not be that obvious.

2) In this interval—the only place in the enneagram where it occurs—there are two parallel routes between the points. One is the 5→7 path along the circle, a process proceeding outwardly though time at its own tempo; and the other is the inner line 5→7, which is an instantaneous psychological parallel and can vastly confuse the issue.

3) There is the involvement of point-six, which comes from a different level altogether and provides a shock to go through, analogous to the action of point-three on the 2→4 interval, only this time the polarity is reversed and the action is much more subtle, therefore easily misunderstood.

4) The 5→7 interval (point-six in particular) has been dubbed in Gurdjieffian terminology the "Harnel-Aoot" or the "disharmonizing mdnel-in" because of inherent difficulties at this step of the process, as we shall discuss.

It is most likely lawful that I myself, in the writing of this monograph, am feeling a disharmony at precisely this point. It is manifesting as a confusion about how to proceed in light of the above-described complexity. I wish to make this account clear and coherent for the reader, and yet as one might surmise, this interval is perhaps the most confusing and multifaceted part of the octave; and it is here that I begin to doubt my own understanding and my ability to transmit what I do know about this stopinder, that is, to transmit it in a way that will make sense, be consistent, and approach to even some semblance of an objective description.

The pitfalls at this point are hesitation and indecision. At point-five one has achieved a result, but it is an unstable position. The effort here is to continue. "Begin. Continue," as the Zen saying goes. By analogy suppose a mountain climber, who after scaling a steep wall finally comes to a slim ledge where he can rest. But if the ledge contains loose rock or if it is very late in the day and if he tarries too long, he would be in real trouble.

In the healing octave, if one stops treatment at point-five or shortly after—either by imagining that "now it will get better by itself," or by being discouraged that the progress is so slow—regression is likely, because it is a fragile and unstable stage of the process. However, when the patient's discouragement is a result of feeling the need for some different type of therapy to increase the rate of their healing, in that case, it is a time either to experiment or to add new modalities. For difficult cases it sometimes takes more than one type of therapy in order for healing to continue.

In my case, with the writing of this chapter, I don't see exactly how to proceed, but if I were to wait too long to decide, I would lose the continuity and the thread of it. The rhythm would be disrupted, "the time would go out of it" and this manuscript might easily end up on the shelf with a few others that were never finished either.

Strictly speaking however, point-five in a writing project comes after the rough draft has been completed, after there has been a result. Then the manuscript needs to be rewritten, proof-read, edited, prepared for publication, etc. In this case, I am nowhere near that point at present. But perhaps I am feeling the disharmonizing effects simply by attempting to write about this stopinder. After all, there are octaves within octaves.

So it feels now that the next topic to be discussed should be just this disharmonizing phenomenon, the Harnel-Aoot.

The way Gurdjieff originally explained it in *Beelzebub's Tales*, was that this disharmonizing interval is the consequence of the asymmetry of the fundamental cosmic laws, which has a correlate in the musical octave. Specifically, the Mi-Fa interval is longer than the space between the other notes (in terms of the frequency or pitch) and the Si-Do interval is shorter. The consequence is the disharmony in the Sol-La interval. It should be stated that the Sol-La interval is the same length as the others, for example Do-Re, Re-Mi, etc. The disharmony comes from the innate characteristics of the octave as a whole. (See Figure 6-1 on page 73, which shows this part of the enneagram.)

I don't understand why this disharmony must be so in a theoretical sense, again, any more than I understand the basis of the physical laws of the universe. But observed in a practical, experiential way, the Harnel-Aoot can be identified in every process and project at this exact stage. One picture that may help to visualize this is to imagine an eight step staircase made of some hard plastic that is all one unit. Then imagine that the riser between the third and fourth step was stretched and the one between the seventh and eighth step was compressed. This change would effect the integrity of the rest of the structure and likely cause some strain and tension somewhere in the middle; maybe at the fifth step.

Gurdjieff used the word "disharmonizing" perhaps because of his musical background; I used the words "strain" and "tension" in the example because I am a doctor who relates to musculo-skeletal problems. However I think the ideas are analogous. In fact, in my experience working on patient's spines I often notice that if a patient has a compression of a vertebra in their neck combined with a twist or rotation in the low back (which may have a lengthening effect on one side), there will often be a painful tension somewhere in the middle. Most chiropractors take this phenomenon for granted, and call these consequences in the middle of the spine, "compensations."

By the way, in these examples of the spine and the rigid staircase, we are considering the enneagram not of a process but of a seven-aspected phenomenon, like the musical octave. However, in the enneagram of a process, the underlying laws should be the same as well.

An example of an actual process will illustrate how disharmony happens at this stage. This example relates to an experience I had building a house a few years ago. In this particular process, point-five is reached after the frame of the house is completed, the roof is in place, and one can visualize in three dimensions instead of two what the house will look like, at least when it gets to point-seven.

It was a shock to observe at this point that everything didn't go exactly according to plan, that the plans themselves weren't exactly what we had in mind—which caused friction with the architect, and that the subcontractors had made some mistakes—which caused disharmony with the builders. And then there was the building inspector from the county who needed to examine the structure at this stage before allowing the builders to proceed further. The diligent inspectors always seem to find some little detail in the construction that doesn't conform to their arcane "code," and must be redone. At this step the experience can be one of frustration and even despair—to look at the skeletal structure, overwhelmed by the amount of work and expense still ahead, and not able to believe that it could ever be finished, and yet not be able to go back.

John Bennett, in his book, *Talks on Beelzebub's Tales* sees the Harnel-Aoot in a very similar way:

"In climbing a mountain, one must reach the point at which there is no feeling that it is possible to reach the top and no feeling that one can return to the bottom. Once that point is passed, no matter how hard the going is, one has the confidence of getting there in the end."[1]

Actually, I have had that kind of experience climbing a mountain in Northern New Mexico in the mid 1970"s. After walking six miles up a steep canyon and arriving at the base of the peak itself, I gazed up at the

1 Bennett, *Talks on Beelzebub's Tales*, p.57.

vertical mass looming ahead and in the vernacular of today's youth: I was like "we have to go up there? No way."

To complete the climb seemed like having to start over, except from the point of being half-exhausted. But when one is so close to a peak, there is an optical illusion that makes it seem bigger and taller than it actually is. Likewise, when one is immersed in a building project, and comes to the Harnel-Aoot, the work looming ahead, although daunting, may seem magnified out of proportion.

In the example of building the house, my wife and I were able to correct all the minor problems, persevere through the later stages of the process and eventually live in a beautiful new house.

There have been other building projects however, that I have been aware of over the years, that have led to divorces, lawsuits, delays, and/or abandonment of the project altogether, and it is often the Harnel-Aoot that was the initiator of the disaster.

To reiterate, the central idea is that in any building project, whether it is a house, hotel, a bridge, or a barn that is being built, there inevitably comes that point in the process after the initial result is achieved, where it is observed that either something has gone awry or the goal seems impossibly far away.

The Harnel-Aoot occurs in every process; and one factor that helps people get through this difficulty is the accomplishment of reaching point-five itself. When there is an initial result, and one can visualize how further work, or treatment, in the case of the healing process, needs to go, then there is hope that the process can continue to completion. This is the hope of cancer patients who, although weak and debilitated, achieve a remission after their first round of chemotherapy or other treatment; it is the hope of heart-attack victims who survive and begin to recover, the hope of asthmatics after they can breathe again after treatment for an acute attack.

This is also a time for experimentation, as I mentioned earlier. The 5→7 interval is a different direction than 4→5, another deflection of the octave; and what worked to bring a patient to point-five may not be sufficient or appropriate for the patient to reach point-seven.

For example, chiropractic adjustments may totally relieve a person's neck pain, but if the pain returns a few days or weeks after every adjustment, something different may be needed to reach point-seven, for example a traction device to restore the curvature in the cervical spine, cranial adjustments to restore the functioning of the supporting tissues, or perhaps deep work on the musculature. For different patients, one or another of these adjuncts have often been necessary for them to reach point-seven.

Another factor in helping patients go through the Harnel-Aoot is the shock of going through point-six as we shall see in the next chapter.

## Chapter 6
# Point Six and the 5→7 Inner Line

Point-six, like point-three, is part of the triangle superimposed over the enneagram circle. This is the second node where the fundamental laws of the universe intersect. At point-three in the healing octave, as we discussed, the world acts on the ill person and allows them or prevents them from finding the help that they need. The world is active and the patient is passive. At point-six there is the opposite polarity, the recovering person is now active and the world—their surroundings, are passive and yielding. In other words, at point-three the world acts on me, and at point-six I act on the world.

This is the stage where the person has recovered enough to return to their daily routine, as it were, from their previous illness or incapacitation. Now the world has to adapt to them. This can be seen clearly by patients being released from a hospital or recovering from a trauma. Almost always, there is a period where they will need some care, either from relatives, friends, or professionals. The person "coming back" is causing the world to adapt to them. It may be as straightforward as domestic help, or a little more complicated, like an employer having to make some changes so that his rehabilitating employee can do "modified work" until he is physically capable of performing his former duties.

There is an example of this phenomenon from my practice, an interesting case history that occurred about ten years ago. The patient in question had recently moved to Central Oregon with her family from a farming community in the San Joaquin Valley of California, in the land of giant agribusiness. She was now suffering from depression, had tried two or three anti-depressants, and they were not helping her at all. The part that was odd to me was that in that part of California amidst all the farm chemicals and pollution, she was healthy. It was only after she had been in the clean, dry climate of the high desert, which she really liked, that the depression set in. There was nothing amiss in her domestic or emotional life that could explain it. The only clue was that her husband owned a small-engine repair shop, and she did the bookkeeping for the business, sitting in a cubicle in the shop. I ordered a hair mineral analysis and found that her vanadium levels were off the chart (extremely high vanadium levels are very rare). Her husband sharpened chainsaws and lawnmower blades every day, and she had been breathing in the metallic dust and happened to be very sensitive to it. Vanadium, which is used to harden steel, is a nutrient in microgram quantities but is toxic in milligram amounts, and the larger amounts can cause depression.

After two or three weeks on a metal detoxification regimen, her depression was completely gone. Her husband however, had to reconfigure his shop, and build a separate ventilated area for her office (her point-six experience). Then she was eventually back to being her normal self again.

There is also a more subtle aspect of passing through point-six. Every gravity-center that is experienced in this octave, every interval that is crossed, as we said, brings about a transformation. In the healing octave, as in any "ascending" octave, the energies become finer and more ethereal as we ascend the left side of the enneagram circle.

As a dysfunctional organism is gradually restored to health through the efforts of the patient and the doctor together, the patient going through these changes is himself/herself transformed in some real way at each step. Part of the shock at point-six is the "world" reacting and having to relate to this transformed person. There will be changes in the behavior of the people around the recovering person. Perhaps they will be more attentive, more interested in who this new person is, that is, how they have changed. From the patient's point of view, there is sometimes a shock of feeling the kindness and caring of people toward them that evokes a gratitude and an energy that may assist their continued healing.

In any case, at point-six the "world" has to react in some way to the patient's needs, and this interaction can provide the shock needed to reach point-seven, a place where the recovered person can again function without overt symptoms.

Point-six has a similar quality in the octave of spiritual-development. There is a fine example of this in the movie, *Meetings with Remarkable Men*. I am referring to the scene where Gurdjieff and Prince Lubachevsky are sitting together just outside the Sarmoung Monastery, before the prince is about to depart. He tells Gurdjieff:

> "Stay here until you have a force in you that nothing can destroy. Then go back into the world and measure yourself constantly against forces that will show you your place."

The new initiate's return to the world is a classic point-six experience. Their intention and activity will collide with the resistance provided by the world, and either carry them to point-seven or not.

Those of us who have worked in spiritual groups have a rudimentary taste of this experience after a period of intense work at, for example, a week-long retreat isolated from the frantic rhythm of today's world, usually on some group-owned property in the countryside.

When the retreat is over the participants must rejoin the outer world, transformed in some small but real way that changes the energy they project, that changes their conduct toward other people, and thus invites anyone who comes in contact with them to feel that change and respond to it. For the participants themselves the initial shock of being relatively awake in a sleeping world can be overwhelming and almost too much to bear.

There is another element of point six that is important to include here, that is more subtle and difficult to describe. Whenever, in a process, one comes to those special places, that is points three, six, and nine, then one is connected at those moments with a greater cosmic law. At point six it is not just about getting to point seven and continuing one's healing process, although that is a major part of it, but there can an experience of being in touch with something greater than oneself, this fundamental cosmic law, the Law of Three. The interface between one's process and this law provides a shock, that enables one, for this moment, to be in touch with a larger part of the process. The whole healing process can be thought of as sacred, in the American Indian sense of, "in a sacred manner we live," but if there is one place where this feeling can be especially felt, it is at point six. It is here, when one's health is improving to the stage where one can almost function normally again, when one does not yet feel like "themself" but can see that coming on the horizon, that it is possible to see the whole process from an entirely different perspective, to perhaps feel an intense gratitude for being able to be a functioning part of this amazing universe again, or just for *being* itself.

The final aspect of this 5→6→7 journey to be discussed is the 5→7 inner line.

It is interesting and instructive that on the right side of the enneagram circle the subject, upon making the commitment to a particular healing system at point-two, gets a glimpse very far ahead to being in a restored state of health (2→8 inner line). As Prince Lubachevsky told the young Gurdjieff in a earlier part of the movie, *Meetings*, "At the beginning this kind of help is needed."

That is, one receives a vision of what is possible, which provides enough energy and motivation to do the work around the circle to make it happen.

However (back to the healing octave), even when one has done some of the work getting to point-five, a place where "the worst is over," then one is only given a glimpse of the next step, point-seven, the place where one can at least function again without pain or disability. At first glance, it may not seem "fair" that the universe functions in this way; that is, that one should be given the vision of reaching a lofty goal early on (the 2→8 inner line), then after much struggle only be given a view slightly ahead (the 5→7 inner line). But upon further pondering, it seems right that what one really needs at point-five is simply to be inspired by that vision of point-seven, to gain the faith that they can indeed pass through the Harnel-Aoot if they persevere. For example, patients that have been suffering with pain for quite a long time arrive at point-five somewhat improved, maybe still having good days and bad days. At that stage all they wish for is to be free of pain. They are not yet concerned with a higher level of health.

A pitfall relating to the 5 →7 inner line is connected to the fact that a fantasy can be mistaken for a vision. There is a fine line between a vision, which is a real premonition—an insight that has perhaps materialized from a higher plane—and a fantasy, that comes from imagination or wishful thinking.

On the left side of the circle as I noted earlier, there are finer energies at play at each succeeding step, but one can easily be mislead by imposters of these subtle energies. To appreciate this distinction, consider the fine line between the personality of a guru and that of a crazy person. The former delights in spontaneous and unpredictable action as a conscious choice, where as the latter acts without awareness and with very little control over random impulses that appear in his/her mind. But to a casual, uninitiated observer they both may appear equally crazy. In reality, the spiritual master and the psychotic are on opposite sides of the spectrum. Likewise, there is a fine line between the appearance of a vision and a fantasy, although they too are almost opposites.

The consequence of a patient stuck at point-five, who is unwilling to continue treatment, and imagines that they are healed enough to reengage in their life, is that the inner line 5→7 can become a triad of 5→7→1, and the patient may have to start all over again. (See Figure 6-1 on page 74.)

Re-injury, relapse, or aggravation of the problem is often one misstep away, for example, during a stressful day at work. The consequence of a regression at this point could be a fall all the way back to point-one, and then the patient would face the same challenges a second time. The above scenario is a bit like the childhood game, "chutes and ladders," only much more real.

The "slide" back to point-one often happens to compulsive workers who literally can't endure a life without constant activity, constant doing. Sometimes their justification is the notion that they can't afford not to work; sometimes they have the illusion that the world can't function without them; and occasionally it is simply an obsession to always be busy and productive.

A variation of this latter trait was the downfall of a long-time patient of mine a few years ago. At the time she was undergoing medical treatment for breast cancer, and I was treating her for back pain, and giving her some nutritional advice. After that period she was fine for a year or two, but eventually her tumor returned, and when I next saw her the medical doctors had given up on her and she was in pretty bad shape. As a last resort, I told her about a natural cancer remedy that was available at the time, and she obtained a bottle and took it according to the directions. By the second or third day after taking this elixir, she felt 90% better, and had most of her energy back. Having all this energy, she couldn't sit still and against everyone's advice spent a whole day cleaning her house. Unfortunately, this family had to put their house up for sale to pay the medical bills, and a clean house does facilitate a sale. But the next day after all that exertion, she was exhausted again and it took another bottle of this elixir and another week before she was able to function. But when she started feeling better the second time, the same cycle repeated and this time the remedy (which is quite expensive) wasn't sufficient. Discouragement set in and she died a couple of months later.

On the 5→6→7 journey, feeling good again can be a blessing, but it can also be a curse, if one isn't able to make a corresponding change in one's habit patterns.

The 5→7→1 inner line phenomenon also happens to vain optimists whose nature is to believe that

    a)   no matter what, everything will be OK, and that

    b)   since they're special, they can violate natural laws (a little bit) and get away with it.

I have to confess that when I was a beginning pupil at Two Rivers Farm, we were presented with a long list of chief features[1], and the one that struck a chord and rang true for me was "optimistic self-love." Personally, I have suffered through this 5→7→1 slide more times than I can remember, and it was always because I had the illusion when I reached point-five or at least before I arrived at point-seven, that, "now I'm OK," and that because I am above the law, I can get away with some extra work, or with eating suspect foods, or staying up late exhausting myself, or getting too emotionally involved with injustices, etc., before I was really better. There

---

1 See *In Search of the Miraculous*, p 266-8, for a discussion about chief feature.

was also the (mistaken) belief that these activities would have no negative consequences.

I'm one of those people who has needed to repeat this kind of experience over and over many times, until I have been to able to be awake at the crucial moment. If one wakes up before the momentum of the activity has dissolved one's intention, it is possible to prevent a complete regression of the dysfunction.

Now, in my life I feel like a cat with nine lives that has squandered eight of them. There is no longer any alternative but to go through this part of the process as consciously as possible.

I sincerely hope the reader will learn from these mistakes, and not have to reinvent the wheel if you find yourself in a similar situation.

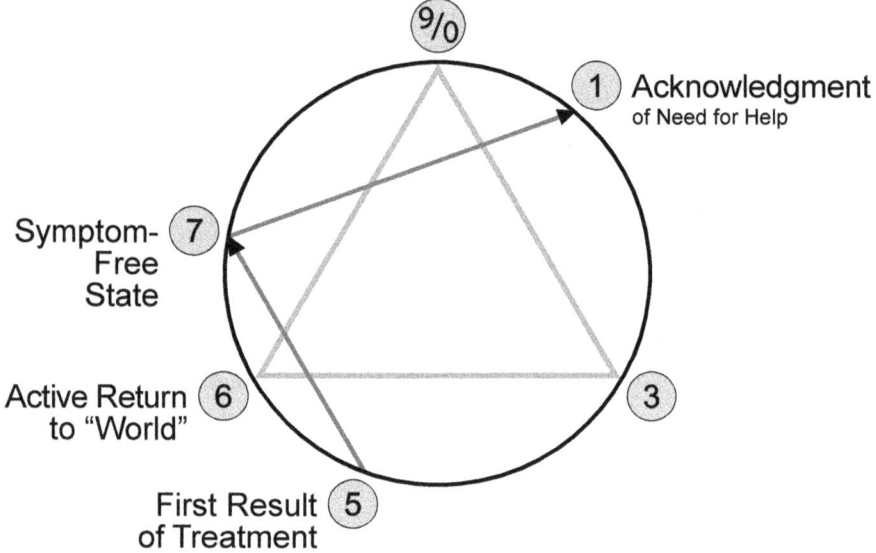

**Figure 6-1,** *Partial Enneagram focusing on the 5→6→7 Interval and associated Inner Lines*

The 5→6→7 interval (the fifth stopinder, also called the "Harnel-Aoot"), is that "disharmonized" part of the process where the patient arises from his or her "sick-bed," in a manner of speaking, and again must confront his or her surroundings, only this time as an active force, and the "world" adapts to or receives the recovering patient. For the healing to continue, usually some change in the treatment regime is necessary during this phase. Also, the 5→7 inner line can allow the patient to imagine they are better before they actually are, in which case there is the danger of regressing all the way back to point-one (the 7→1 inner line).

## Chapter 7
# Point Seven

When one approaches point-seven on the enneagram of healing, one is finally, for the time being, free of symptoms. However, there is a distinction between being temporarily free of symptoms and being healthy. Being free of symptoms is a stage one goes through on the way to a more optimal state of health. This is an idea that is sometimes difficult to get across to patients, especially those who are impatient to be well, and finished with their distracting difficulties.

The problem is that the dysfunction in a human body can progress to a certain extent before a person is aware of it. Then there may be symptoms, such as pain, digestive upsets, dizziness, coughing, skin lesions, fever, difficulty breathing, fatigue, or any of hundreds of other symptoms that one can easily perceive. Likewise, as the body heals, these symptoms may subside and even disappear well before the dysfunction is finally resolved in terms of the complete restoration of cellular integrity, and the return of the organs to normal functioning.

As diagnosticians, we now have incredibly sensitive ways to determine subtleties of dysfunction. Traditional Chinese doctors using their special form of pulse diagnosis were cognizant of these sub-clinical abnormalities even in ancient times.

A condition is "sub-clinical" when the patient is not aware of it. But it is possible for the doctor to observe the dysfunction through trained observation or sensitive testing. In chiropractic, we take this phenomenon almost for granted. We are accustomed to observing a patient's posture and skeletal features, for example, and seeing various asymmetries and structural abnormalities of which the patient is not aware, and that predisposes them to specific kinds of injuries or degenerative changes.

At point-seven, the patient has reached a symptom-free status, but their skeletal structure, and/or biomechanics, and/or body chemistry, and/or emotional life are not yet back to normal; they have not yet reached a dynamic equilibrium that can withstand the stresses with which people are often faced.

How does one experience point-seven?

For me, the situation has been as follows: One day or hour, I will wake up and realize that I have been breathing normally for a while, that my energy level is adequate, that I haven't needed any special medicines or remedies lately.

As one approaches point-seven, one tends to forget about the healing process, as one again becomes immersed in their daily routine, and as the rate of change in one's condition continues to slow down until the day-to-day changes become imperceptible. This is especially true for people like me, who at early periods of their life have been healthy and free from significant dysfunction for long periods. During those earlier times I forgot that I was an asthmatic.

This variety of the experience of point-seven also happens to patients recovering from chronic back, shoulder, neck, hip pain, etc. There comes a point when they have been back to work for a while, still continuing treatment, but not as frequently, and one day they realize that their pain is practically gone, they are functioning normally, and they sometimes affirm, "I've got my life back."

In my own recent experience there is a secondary reaction to this kind of realization, which is for a time to be very, very careful, like walking on eggshells, as the saying goes. The caution I exercise is a result of going through this part of the process many times, as I mentioned at the end of the previous chapter. When I remember the difficult struggle to ascend from point-five, and also assimilate the help that comes from the 7→1 inner line—which allows me to recall and revisit the depths of point-one—I begin to guard my health as if hoarding a cache of precious stones, whenever I again become aware that I have reached point-seven. This caution, as I noted, is mostly a result of learning from past experience. In my earlier life, and for certain other types of people, as soon as they reach point-seven, they proceed with reckless abandon.

Point-seven—like point-five in this regard—is not yet a stable position. Stability comes at point-eight, but to ascend to that level requires another new kind of effort. However when one reaches point-seven, where the symptoms have abated, and in some cases when one imagines that everything is back to normal, back to "roses, roses"—like it might have been when they were a late teenager—this is when things begin to slide downhill.

In my case, when I have grown accustomed to feeling "normal" again, the "walking on eggshells" phase fades away quickly, and if I don't begin to make particular new efforts (that I will discuss later), then little by little, unconsciously, the old habits come back and a downhill octave commences.

The old habits that impede healing—specifically for the 7→8 movement—are different for different people, but some of them are:

1) An irresistible urge to prematurely return to full-time work again, or even worse, to work harder than before in order to get "caught up with one's life" as with the breast cancer patient.

2) A habit of insufficient sleep, which often goes along with the first habit mentioned. Sleep is a great healer, especially at this stage. It is matter of energy economy. The alert and working brain uses a tremendous amount of the body's resources. When the brain is quiet, much of this energy can be channeled into healing. When one is in an intense stage of healing, there will be a natural urge for sleep which can be actualized only if the conditions of our lives allow us to surrender to it.

3) A habit of dietary imbalance. For a great number of people, various foods cause allergic, hyper-sensitivity, or inflammatory reactions in the body. The foods people crave the most, and the ones to which they are emotionally attached, are often the worst offenders. Being passive and uninvolved in one's food choices in this era can lead to disaster by itself. I refer the reader to Michael Pollan's books for useful information on this subject.

4) A reversion to energy-draining emotional habits, which tend to re-emerge when one's health again increases, and often result from the inability to endure the unpleasing, insensitive, or selfish manifestations of other people in one's sphere. Allowing oneself to squander newly regained energy in anger, indignation, resentments, etc. at this stage definitely prevents further progress and can even catalyze the downward slide back to point-one.

There are two metaphors that illuminate the point-seven experience from other perspectives: The first is that of a salmon swimming up the river to return home to spawn. Point-seven is like a wide, slow moving place in the river, say below a cataract or small waterfall, an eddy below some white water, where the salmon can rest for a while before summoning the strength to continue moving upstream against a more formidable current and more danger. If the salmon can't hurdle this obstacle, or figuratively goes to sleep and forgets its aim, it will drift back down the river with the current. From the river mouth to the first cataract, which is like the 5→7 leg of the journey, the river is wide and deep and the current is gentle. But then there is a new kind of effort required for the salmon to find it's way above the obstacles, and to reach its spawning grounds. Without that effort it would eventually slide backward.

The second metaphor concerns spiritual development. After many years of inner efforts, one may reach a place where one has a functional knowledge of the practices and the theory of one's lineage, is able to maintain a sense of presence, of being here, now, for short periods of time, and even assist younger pupils and answer their questions. But if these results are not yet "crystallized," not a permanent part of the seeker's being, they can still be lost. Like the salmon, when one stops making efforts, one slips downhill. In both cases, as I mentioned earlier, point-seven is an unstable place. One can't stay there for long. Either one makes further efforts and ascends toward point-eight or one forgets and slides back toward point-one. If one doesn't continue going forward the current irresistibly pulls one backward.

In the octave of the digestion and transformation of food that Gurdjieff described in the chapter Purgatory of *Beelzebub's Tales*[1], point-seven is the level of "piandjoehary," a finer energy which is associated

---
1 Gurdjieff, *Beelzebub's Tales* pp. 786-792.

with the cerebellum. It is interesting to note that the roots of the word, cerebellum, mean "seat of war." As Gurdjieff explains it, there is a conflict here between opposing forces:

> "Just these same substances in beings... have the free possibility of giving... results not similar but 'opposite to each other.'
> "That is why, in respect of these being-substances, the beings themselves must always be very, very much on their guard in order to avoid undesirable consequences for their entire whole."[2]

One way of interpreting this oft-quoted dictum is in the discussion I've given above. If one makes efforts they will move forward toward point-eight; if they stop or only imagine they are working, they will descend downward toward point-one. There is no middle ground, no maintaining a status quo. One can either ascend or descend—results opposite to each other.

Another way to understand this idea of "results opposite to each other," has to do with the function of these fine energies or "substances" acting on the brain.

Tetartoehary, at point-five in the food octave, is the energy of logical, literal thinking associated with parts of the cerebral cortex. When some of this energy is transformed into the finer substance piandjoehary, the new function is "form-thinking" or visualization. But now there are two opposite possibilities, because form-thinking can also manifest as negative imagination, which yields results opposite of being able to visualize, for example, a desired outcome, and working toward it. The latter would lead a person toward point-eight. The former, say picturing oneself failing, or picturing oneself being a victim of circumstances that absolutely prevent achieving a higher level of health, or perhaps constant worry that one's symptoms will return—these negative uses of piandjoehary can become a self-fulfilling prophecy, and therefore lead to an "opposite result."

By the same token, the delusion that one has already reached their goal also leads to these opposite results.

---
2 Gurdjieff, *Beelzebub's Tales*, p. 791.

In terms of the healing process, point-seven is where, as I mentioned, there is the pitfall that one can imagine that they are already healed. The nagging symptoms have in fact abated, and therefore it might seem that no further effort would be needed. So the attitude of "back to life as usual" may begin to prevail. But as the popular saying goes, "if you do what you have always done, you will get what you've always got."

When point-seven is reached, it can be irresistibly tempting, for example, for the alcoholic, who was abstaining while recovering from a health problem, to have just one small drink, or for the person who has recovered from a recent heart-attack to revert back to their old artery-clogging diet.

The downhill octave (the 7→1 inner line) starts very gradually but soon picks up momentum and reaches a tipping-point, a point of no return, where one falls to a bottom and has to begin again.

An unexpected source of information about the nature of point-seven can be found in the Lord's Prayer. When the phrases of the prayer are arranged around the enneagram circle in order, point-six and seven occur around the phrase "Lead us not into temptation, but deliver us from evil."

Did the authors of this prayer know about the enneagram? Or did they understand in an intuitive way that there is an inevitable stage in a disciple's development just before they enter the "kingdom," when they will be tempted? Evil, in a broad esoteric sense, means those influences that lead one away from their aim. Part of the effort both to reach point-seven and to ascend from point-seven is to resist temptation. We have already discussed this somewhat in terms in the need to resist old habits.

There is also another remarkable connection between the Lord's Prayer and the healing octave. I will digress briefly to explore this further:

I realized that for the Lord's Prayer enneagram, point-four would be, "Forgive us our trespasses," and point-five, "As we forgive those who trespass against us." (See Figure Ap-3 on page 120, for an enneagram of the Lord's Prayer.)

In other words, at point-four we ask for forgiveness, and by the time we reach point-five, we are the ones doing the forgiving. In this light, work on forgiveness is the crux of the whole prayer. This relates to the healing octave in a big way because emotional healing in many cases underlies, that is provides a foundation for physical healing.

In my practice, I've seen many patients who need to engage in the work of forgiveness. Two types of people come to mind:

1) Those who have been through divorces, sometimes years earlier, and still harbor anger, even hatred toward their ex-spouse. Strong, chronic, negative emotions, even when they are partially repressed, rob energy from the immune system and healing in general as I alluded to earlier. Whether these long-standing resentments cause physical illness or merely are a factor that perpetuates it, is a moot point. The fact is that the negative emotion and the physical illness are frequently associated with each other.

2) the other category of patients who would need work on forgiveness are those who had been abused as children—either sexually, physically, or psychologically/emotionally. According to current estimates this category may represent more than 50% of adults in America in the first decade of the 21st century. Any kind of deep-seated trauma in one's past, especially if it has never been self-examined, that is, in therapy or by some kind of inner Work, very often leads to one type of physical ailment or another. I have verified this over and over in my practice. There comes a time, upon ascending from point-seven, where one needs to confront these emotional devils lurking under the surface of one's consciousness if there is to be any hope of a stable, more optimal state of health.

In Dr. Bach's words,

> Suffering [with a health problem] is a corrective to point out a lesson which by other means we have failed to grasp, and can never be eradicated until that lesson is learned. [3]

In my own case, I grew up with a father who had an explosive, unpredictable temper that erupted occasionally, and who was also mildly abusive in the sense of criticism, ridicule, and humiliation. In all fairness, these episodes were infrequent and on the whole I grew up in a secure

---
3 Bach, *Heal Thyself* (pp 8-9).

environment in the suburbs with two parents who did care about me and were always there. But as a child, it was sometimes difficult emotionally, because I never knew when he was going to be a father-protector or when he was going to be a hostile enemy. And as he grew older his emotional state deteriorated, his health worsened, and he incurred additional suffering over the fact that as an adult, I had no interest in visiting him other than the bare minimum dictated by family obligation. Eventually, however, there came a point in my study of esoteric teachings when I understood that it was necessary to forgive my father even though he had died several years earlier. An ongoing inability to forgive him, even after his demise, would become an obstacle to my own evolution, and my health.

My first attempts at this were mainly to affirm, "I forgive you".

But I know now that a declaration like this which comes from the ordinary mind, has about as much weight, energetically, as a New Year's resolution. And from further pondering I now cognize that point-four in this regard does have to come before point-five. In other words, first I have to ask to be forgiven. When I remember and re-experience the times that I was particularly insensitive and inconsiderate of my father as a older child and a teenager, a feeling of remorse arises, however fleeting. Remorse, our link to a buried conscience, is connected to the heart. It is an emotion, a positive emotion. When I ask for forgiveness in the aftertaste of this feeling of remorse a connection is made with my heart, and somehow this lifts the whole experience to a higher part of myself, and gives me a reference for how it feels to really engage in the act of forgiveness.

I wonder whether the last words of Jesus on the crucifix (according to Matthew), embodies these principles:

"Forgive them Father, for they know not what they do."

He did not say, "I forgive them," but "Forgive them Father."

We know what the more literal interpretation of "Father" is, but perhaps on a symbolic level, it has to do with the highest part of ourselves, the part that is the potential master. Forgiveness needs to come from the "father", the highest, most refined part, not the ordinary mind.

But even this more conscious work on forgiveness needs to be revisited many times before it penetrates into all the interstices of one's mind, and finally dissolves the remnants of anger and resentment, so that a more sincere form of compassion can emerge. Then the ascent from point-seven on the healing octave is on a firmer footing.

CHAPTER 8

# The 7→8 interval

One essential feature of the interval or stopinder between point-seven and point-eight is change, in the sense of transformation. We just spoke of a change of heart in terms of the work on forgiveness. There are also other transformations related to the heart that are helpful if not necessary to cross this space.

For example, the sense of entitlement that I deserve to be healthy and deserve not to have to suffer, can be transformed into a gratitude for what I do have. That in itself saves a huge amount of energy that can be used for healing.

Another example of an emotional transformation that can facilitate the arrival at point-eight is the change of attitude from resignation into hope. In other words, a change from feeling stuck at a certain point and being resigned to it –into acquiring the hope that one's situation can improve to the next level. In fact one benefit of learning about the enneagrammatic nature of the healing process is to connect with that sense of hope.

There are physical changes that need to happen as well, on the way to point-eight. At point-seven one is free of symptoms, but lacking in reserves of energy and vitality. The organs have perhaps not regained their full function, and the muscles may have not regained their previous strength. It is a fragile state that can be disrupted with even a small amount of stress. The available energy for leading a normal life can be depleted unexpectedly. So the new efforts to ascend from point-seven entail a strengthening of the body and a building up of reserves of energy, like filling a mostly empty reservoir.

In order to do this it is necessary to make a change in one's habits—to create a time and place each day (or several days a week) for some kind of discipline or practice. This interval represents not the path to get well, that was 5→7, but the path to achieve a more stable and durable quality of health, which after a long recovery from an illness or an injury requires a different kind of effort. Here I will repeat the popular saying, "If you do what you've always done, you get what you've always got." The corollary to this saying is, "One definition of insanity is doing what you've always done and expecting a different result."

One can see the tragic consequences of the popular sayings quoted above on the national level in the results of the so-called "war on drugs" or the "war on poverty," which have been plodding along in the same way for over forty years now, and both the drug problem and the poverty problem in America are worse than ever before. No one in a position of authority seems to have the capability or the courage to suggest a change of course. Fortunately, the ability to make a change in one's personal habits is more possible than a change in an entrenched and corrupt bureaucracy involving tens or hundreds of thousands of people. Again, at this stage something different—a new effort—is needed.

The interval of point-seven to point-eight requires the willingness to undermine one's self-imposed limitations, and often this becomes possible only after a new way of thinking is developed.

By analogy, in the octave of spiritual development, there is a remarkable example of the creative effort needed to ascend through the 7→8 interval in the Third Series of Gurdjieff's writings, *Life is Real Only Then, When "I Am"*:

> " In my past life .... I could attain almost anything within the limit of man's possibilities .... for instance, the development of the power of my thoughts had been brought to such a level that by only a few hours of self-preparation I could from a distance of tens of miles kill a yak .... at the same time in

spite of all my desires and endeavors, I could not succeed in 'remembering myself' in the process of my general common life with others ...."[1]

The above quote is a small part of a self-examination Gurdjieff initiated in himself while recovering from one of his bullet wounds in a "salutary" and paradisiacal oasis on the edge of the Gobi desert. Upon continuing his profound meditation on his dilemma (which really is the problem faced by all who attempt to Work on themselves—the inability to remember ourselves more often in spite of our best efforts), he finally had another epiphany:

> "Thinking and thinking, I came to the conclusion that if I should intentionally stop utilizing the exceptional power in my possession which had been developed by me consciously... then there must be forced out of me such a reminding source. Namely the power based upon strength in the field of 'hanbledzoin,' or, as it would be called by others, the power of telepathy and hypnotism... if consciously I would deprive myself of this grace of my inherency, then undoubtedly always and in everything its absence would be felt.
> "I take an oath to remember never to make use of this inherency of mine and thereby to deprive myself from satisfying most of my vices. In the process of living together with others, this... will always be a reminder for me."[2]

All the elements of the 7→8 journey are contained in Gurdjieff's momentous decision: the need to make a change in order to progress on his path, the necessity of making a serious sacrifice in the process, the masterful surge of creativity that bubbled out, the long and sincere pondering of his situation, and finally the will and the perseverance to make it all come to pass.

---
1 Gurdjieff, *Life is Real Only Then, When "I Am"*, p. 20.
2 Ibid., p. 25.

Attaining point-eight is not something everyone can do in the octave of self-development.

"Many are called, but few are chosen", as the saying goes.

But as Mrs. Staveley noted: "We choose ourselves."

It is a question of will; actually, the willingness to put oneself under a discipline and the willingness to sacrifice what is no longer the top priority.

In the healing octave, reaching point-eight—especially after a chronic illness, serious injury, or addiction to drugs, medications, unhealthy food, etc.—is also very difficult.

As we ascend the left side of the enneagram circle, more and more intention is required at each step. The final step, 8→9, the "intentionally-actualized mdnel-in," whose essence is conscious intentional effort, is the epitome of this principle. But as we can see, 7→8 requires intention also, especially at the outset.

The problem is that when people arrive at point-seven, when they feel they have their life back, there is the illusion, as I have noted, that no further effort is necessary.

For example, one can see this illusion with formerly obese people who have found a way to lose all or most of their excess weight. Statistically, over 95% of these people gain all of their weight back within a year. The reason for this, in terms of the enneagram, is that a different kind of effort with more concerted intention is needed to go from 7→8 than to go from 5→7. This different kind of effort needs to happen after the weight is lost, which unfortunately doesn't stay off by itself. The newly slim person needs to quietly access their situation, in a way analogous but not necessarily as rigorous as the way Gurdjieff undertook this task at the edge of the Gobi desert in 1897. Perhaps a change in lifestyle is needed. Sitting at a desk eight hours each day in front of a computer screen for example, does not lead to good health for anyone, but especially those whose bodies desperately need vigorous physical activity on a daily basis. As Gurdjieff told us again and again in *Beelzebub's Tales*, it is these "abnormal conditions of ordinary life that we ourselves have created," that cause many of our difficulties. So one must seriously question their priorities at this point in the octave.

I will never forget the words of a young Hispanic man from rural New Mexico (sometime in the 1990's) who quit a secure position in a factory in a nearby town, because of the long hours and deficient working conditions:

> "Life is too precious to throw it away just because of a high-paying job."

When a critical mass of people acquires the above attitude, there will be no more jobs that fail to challenge a person in some creative way without beating down their body and spirit.

In my own life, I was able to live that attitude and actually reach point-eight for a few years off and on back in the late 1970's. The intentional part for me happened after my wife and I returned to the US from our travels in 1972. After settling in Boston to complete the last phase of my PhD Work, I couldn't help but notice that people around the city seemed kind of dead compared to the adventurous travelers we had been around for the previous several months. The urbanites that we observed were going through the habitual motions of their repetitive days seemingly on automatic pilot. Mine was not then the perspective of a conscious self-aware individual regarding people asleep to the more objective reality around them and within them. Mine was more the perspective of someone who had just returned from many months of adventure and unpredictability in faraway, unfamiliar countries, where my wits were challenged and my mind was stimulated by new impressions, languages, people, and history on a daily basis.

To again to become engaged in a repetitive, hum-drum life in a drab east-coast city was too much for me to bear. I realized that the happiest and most fulfilling times we had recently experienced were wandering in the wilds of Africa or just being in the mountains far from any city.

So we made the decision to reject the prestigious professional positions we had been offered, and instead drove out West in our VW bug not having a particular destination in mind nor any plan of action when we arrived wherever. However, after only one week on the road, we found and bought forty acres of land at the foot of a mountain in Northern New Mexico in a Pinon-Juniper forest where no one had ever lived before.

It was in retrospect a naive and impractical decision, but on the other hand it restored my health and may have saved my life.

Because of our limited resources and wish to follow the local traditions, we built an adobe house by hand, that is, with our own labor; carved a garden out of ground that was mostly rocks and gravel, walked on long paths through the woods to visit with our neighbors, cut our own firewood, spent 90% of our time outdoors (at 8,000 feet elevation) and generally grew strong and healthy, albeit poor.

This lifestyle started with a decision to make a change, with a new way of thinking, and the courage to reject a late 20th century urban life that would have led to financial security, professional achievement, etc, but that also had been detrimental to my health and emotionally stifling. So, in sum, there was a decision, a sacrifice, and a choice that led to a different kind of life—one that required hard physical work and activity on most days. From 7→8 the relatively conscious choice is made at the beginning, and then one places oneself under the conditions where there is almost no choice but to regain a normal level of health.

In the mid-1990's I had a different kind of 7→8 experience after studying with a Qi Gong master in China for two weeks in 1993. When I returned home I was eager to practice what I had learned, and was diligent in this practice until I returned to China in 1996 with many questions for the teacher, and a need to bring my ability up to another level. When my teacher, Dr. Wan Su Jian, realized who I was one night at dinner during my 1996 trip (he has many students from all over the world) he almost choked on his noodles. My Chi was so much stronger than in 1993 that he didn't even recognize me, because after three years I looked so much younger and more vital.[3]

The difference was that by practicing Qi Gong on a daily basis for those three years my energy gradually increased, so that little by little I was functioning at a higher level and my appearance apparently reflected that. But the change was actually so slow and incremental that I was shocked that people in the group in China in 1996 even noticed a difference.

At this point it might be useful to examine the relationship between Chi (or Qi), the force that underlies our vitality, and what we call the

---

3 See my book, *Healing in China* for the complete story of these trips, and an account of many of the exercises and teachings.

"energy" that powers our metabolism in a physical sense. In other words, how can the increase in this ethereal substance Chi lead to an increase in physical, measurable energy?

This is one of the great mysteries of the world and at present I don't believe anyone does understand in a scientific sense, how something so rarefied as to be almost non-material can be transformed or converted into a physical phenomenon. With the data we have at present it is not explainable; but in my experience it does happen.

My working hypothesis, based on years of pondering and researching this question, is that Chi is a very fine physical substance perhaps composed of photons or electrons, something that is ubiquitous—all around us everywhere—and that we can mobilize and concentrate with specific practices and even with intention. When a large enough quantity of Chi is brought into our bodies it can interact with our bio-molecules, raising them to a higher energy level—much the same way that light activates the electrons in the chlorophyll of plants.

Whether it happens in this way or some altogether different way, the result is the same—one's energy is increased. I have verified that in myself over and over.

The difference between point-seven and point-eight in the enneagram of healing, in a physiological sense, is also largely about energy. When one recovers from an illness or injury or has brought their healing up to point-seven, there may still be in metabolic terms the functioning equivalent to a sedentary person. This is reflected on the cellular level in many ways. One of them is the number of insulin receptors on the surface of each muscle cell, which is a measure of how much fuel the cell can burn. When one has been inactive for a long period of time, the insulin receptors tend to go away. On average an athlete has over a hundred times more insulin receptors per cell than a sedentary person. It is like comparing a lawn mower engine to that of an eight cylinder engine in an automobile. However, when one increases their strength and stamina, not only do the number of insulin receptors increase, but the number of enzymes and other cellular components needed to burn the increased amount of glucose, also proliferate. It is in the nature of our molecular biology that dormant genes will be activated when there is a need for the materials they produce. And not only does each cell have a greater capacity when one has been active and healthy, but of course the body produces much more muscle mass, that is, many times more cells. So by this measure alone, a person at point-eight living a physically active life, has a metabolic capability which translates into strength and endurance that is many, many times greater than the person just reaching point-seven, who nevertheless sometimes "feels like their old self again".

Another physiological measure of the difference between point-seven and eight is bone density. In this case, a single image will convey the difference:

Recently, I had a conversation with an implant dentist who has spent a lot of time over a thirty year career drilling into patient's jawbones. He related to me that drilling into an elite athlete's bone is like trying to drill into metal. It often damages the tiny drill bits. At the other extreme, drilling into the bones of a inveterate "couch potato" is like drilling into styrofoam. There is an initial slight resistance, and then the drill sinks in rapidly as though penetrating a soft, porous material. The dentist insisted that the difference was that dramatic. Of course, this may not be a totally relevant example for 7→8 because bone growth changes that extreme take many years, even decades to manifest, whereas regaining normal health hopefully is a process for most people—depending upon how low their metabolism had previously sunk—that would precede a little more quickly. (In addition, someone with a severe degree of osteoporosis is probably not even close to point-seven).

The above story, however, brings to mind that the 7→8 interval is the place for formerly sedentary (or ill or injured) people to regain their fitness, to get back "in shape," to re-establish their stamina and strength, as well as their sense of themselves as healthy individuals. But regaining one's fitness, as I can well attest, often involves temporary pain and suffering, as does the "healing crisis" in the 4→5 interval. There is a huge obstacle here that is difficult to traverse.

I heard an interesting story a few years ago of a ninety-eight year old man, riddled with the common degenerative conditions of aging, who was complaining to his nephew, a personal trainer. The nephew said to him, "Work with me for two years and I'll have you feeling eighty years old again."

So, at the age of one hundred, the old man felt so much better that he decided to practice throwing the shot put in order to compete at a senior Olympic games event at the Nike campus in Oregon. He proceeded to win his event, throwing the shot nine feet. When he was interviewed by the press afterward, with the usual question of, "How does it feel, etc.?" He answered, "I was just glad I didn't drop it on my foot."

The fact is that when we work with dedication and purpose we surprise even ourselves with what we can achieve. It's the same whether it's sowing a garden or practicing a skill. The rewards are often orders of magnitude greater than the initial efforts.

When one fails to make the inner commitment required to advance to point-eight, believing that no further effort is necessary after the symptoms have abated, the danger, as I have related, is a descent to point-one. Point-seven is a stage where everything can be lost if there is an unwillingness to make the necessary efforts.

Some commentators on the enneagram believe that the inner lines (especially 7→1) represent a kind of eternal recurrence. We repeat and repeat until, as Dr. Bach stated, "The lesson is learned."

In my practice, I witness this phenomenon with older middle-aged patients in physically demanding occupations, whose bodies begin to break down after decades of repetitive stress. This category includes mechanics, construction workers, carpenters, cement contractors, loggers, firefighters, etc. When these types recover from their injuries and find themselves at point-seven, they almost always try to return to what they have done before. I tell them, "You have a choice. You can intentionally make the decision to find some related kind of work that is less physically punishing, or you can wait until you end up in a hospital, and then the choice will be made for you, and it will be fifty times as expensive."

In other words, when a formerly healthy worker nearing the end of his physical capabilities is inwardly active and does make a decision to change careers, he may again reach point-eight. But if he is passive and returns to his occupation by a mechanical kind of momentum, the chances are that he will fall all the way to point-one. I have seen people go in both directions—many times.

Part of the difficulty of avoiding the 7→1 slide is going against the fear of the unknown. For most people it is less scary to return to a familiar and comfortable routine even if it will probably lead to disaster, rather than to face unknown prospects, possible failure, or possible (although unlikely) destitution. Even folk wisdom warns against sudden changes of course, with the old adage, "Don't change horses in midstream."

As the current great recession drags on and the 2012 Mayan mystery deadline looms ever closer, this fear is becoming an issue for large numbers of people, not just those struggling with their healing. People feel the need to make a change but are afraid to take that first step into the unknown, which in our imagination, may be an abyss.

The other difficulty is that the majority of people in this age are estranged from their inner world and their inner knowing; there is no established custom for discovering a new direction in one's life. For example, we have no cultural traditions like the "vision quest" that Native American young adults utilized when they needed guidance for their life's path; or the variation that spontaneously helped Gurdjieff so much at the edge of the Gobi Desert.

So when people arrive at point-seven in their healing, the fear of making a change along with the lack of a source of courage can be a great obstacle to further progress.

It is interesting that there is a similar need at point-two as for the 7→8 interval. One can go beyond point-two only after a decision is made —to seek a specific kind of help. And one can obtain point-eight only if a similar commitment is made: this time the decision to be willing to do what it takes to achieve a sustainable level of health. And these points are connected by the 2→8 line. However, the decision at point-two is borne of a dire need where there is sometimes no viable choice, while the decision allowing one to reach point-eight must come from an active intention, sometimes the result of an understanding that robust health is the foundation of one's life and a prerequisite to fulfill one's other aims.

The decision to strive to reach point-eight can also arise from one's emotional center—the feeling evoked by the awareness of the sacredness and precious quality of life. Emotional impulses give force to one's decisions. So the intention to regain a more stable level of health can come from an understanding or a feeling; in addition, it can even grow out of the body's own wish to be able to move and function the way it did at an earlier time. The intention is of course more potent if the three centers are working together; then there is a much stronger quality of will, discipline and caring for one's real needs.

One final thought on this subject, in regard to the need for normal health to fulfill one's other aims, is that if a person has a higher aspiration, a strong purpose for their life that transcends their own personal agenda, that in itself can become a strong ally. Then the focus is on the Work, not solely on one's health. In this case the body will become "a willing servant" to help the person in their aim; at point-eight one's functioning has risen to the level where one can participate in the transformation of energies that occur on a larger scale. (Figure 8-1 below shows this part of the Healing Enneagram.)

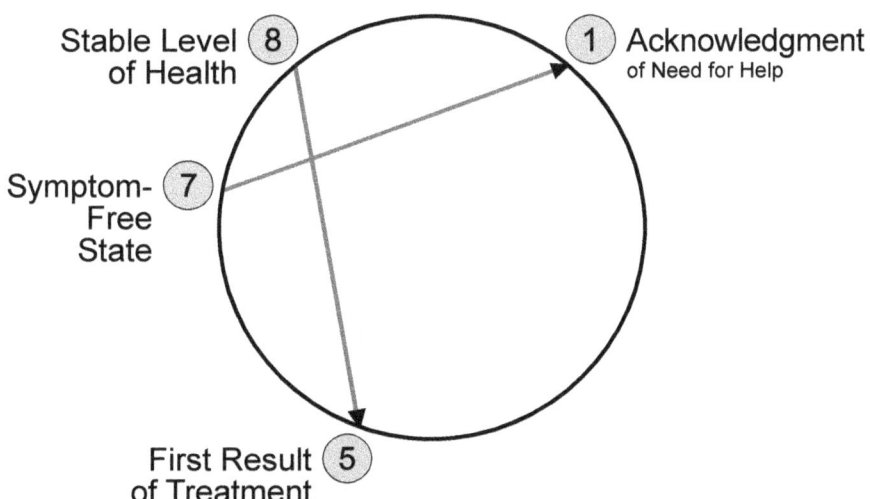

**Figure 8-1,** *Partial enneagram focusing on the 7→8 interval*

The 7→8 interval (or the sixth stopinder) in essence represents the transformation from recovering from an illness or injury, to again being centered in a state of health.

CHAPTER 9
# Point Eight

We have already mentioned some aspects of point-eight in the previous section, but it will be useful to reformulate its primary qualities, which are:

1) a more normal state of health, where there are reserves of energy and

2) a relative stability, or homeostasis (although that latter term might be misleading because point-eight is anything but "static").

What stability means to me in relation to health is a state where one has found a rhythm to one's daily life that is self-sustaining, that can last for a long time, like the rhythm that long distance runners or swimmers find, where each stride or stroke is coordinated with the breathing; the movements of the arms are in synchrony with the movements of the legs, and this engenders—down to the cellular level—an efficiency and coordination of all the parts, a coherence, like a well-tuned machine. In a way this stability or self-sustaining aspect of health is akin to a star in long-term equilibrium, like the sun, where the outward explosive force of the energy-creating nuclear reactions at the center of the sun are exactly balanced by the tremendous inward force of gravity, creating a "steady-state" that can last for billions of years.

This stable state was given to us by nature when we were babies, children, teenagers, even into our twenties and thirties if we were fortunate enough to be born without serious hereditary defects and with parents who were capable and were willing to give us sufficient nutrition, love, security and stimulation. And our state of health could sustain itself if we were lucky enough along the way not to have incurred any disabling injuries nor to have contracted some disease that left lingering after-effects, nor became a victim of some kind of abuse from the outer world. Obviously, there are an almost infinite variety of ways that the body can lose its condition of health and only one way that normal health is expressed—where every part is in working order, and each part works together with all the other parts in a cooperative way.

The human body contains roughly 50-100 trillion cells. If we consider that each one of these cells is essentially a living organism that eats, breathes, eliminates waste, resists infection, makes biological decisions, reproduces, etc., and that we are healthy only when (almost) every one of these little organisms is able to perform a specific function and cooperate with its neighbors for the good of the whole, one can get a picture, a glimpse, of how remarkable it is that this stable state of health can even exist at all. That animals and plants on the earth can live in this state, sometimes for many decades, is certainly one of the greatest miracles of the universe.

Arriving at this state in the context of the healing octave, after recovering from an illness or injury, is a gradual process that can happen in many, almost invisible increments. In fact the whole left side of the enneagram circle becomes increasingly this way as we ascend from point-five. That is, the experiences are more subtle and difficult to describe.

This is in blunt contrast to the right side where there is often a definable, memorable experience at each gravity center: at point-one—the experience of accepting and acknowledging that help is needed; at point-two—the decision of where and how to obtain that help; at point-three—the shock of interaction with the world and the quest to meet that help; and at point-four—the initial contact with the chosen healthcare specialist.

From there it begins to get a little more fuzzy. Although at point-five, people sometimes do see a dramatic improvement after their first "hands-on" treatment for example, or within hours after taking a medicine that happens to be the perfect antidote for their condition. Or they may wake up the next morning after a treatment feeling like their old self again.

But more often the experience of reaching point-five is a slower process, especially with advancing age, severity, or complexity of the condition.

Arriving at point-seven is occasionally a sudden epiphany, but more often a slowly dawning realization; and reaching point-eight is often only noticed in retrospect—after going through an unexpected stress or crisis and realizing that one's health is still intact.

In one sense the points on the left side of the enneagram (points five, seven, eight and nine) represent increasing states of health as well as experiences that mark the arrival at each gravity-center.

In terms of how one feels, the difference between point-seven and eight relates to energy reserves, stamina, endurance; a feeling that once again there is the strength and enthusiasm to take on a new challenge, or return to some kind of work that had become too difficult.

The ability to maintain one's health after going through a difficult or stressful event is in fact, a hallmark of point-eight.

There are many great stories of exploration and survival throughout history, where people have found themselves in situations where they were pushed seemingly passed the limits of human endurance, and managed to return or be rescued—sometimes emaciated, dehydrated, disoriented—but still able to recover.

I recently read an amazing story about a young Polish army officer at the start of World War II who was captured by the Russians, sent to a labor camp in Siberia, and then escaped with six other men after careful planning.[1] They ended up walking many hundreds of miles south out of Siberia in late winter through snow and frozen forests, across Mongolia and the Gobi desert, across Western China, through Tibet, and finally over the Himalayas into safety in Northern India, a total of over 3500 miles. Often they ran out of food, but always kept walking, driven by their imperative for survival and their fear of being recaptured. Sometimes they had only one small meal every three days. Not all of them made it to India, and the ones that did needed a long recovery, but at point-eight—and this is another defining characteristic—the body as I noted, becomes a willing servant, an instrument of the will, and like a faithful horse, will keep going long past the point of exhaustion if the need is critical.

---

1 Slavomir Rawicz, *The Long Walk*.

This latter principle is embodied on a smaller scale in a simple exercise given by John Bennett to his pupils. The class, or group of pupils, stands with arms raised ninety degrees to the side and holds them there for as long as they can, or until the demonstrator indicates to lower them. There comes a point when the arms become so heavy and the shoulder muscles so spent that one is almost compelled let the arms drop. However, if one's will (and wish) are strong enough, and tiny adjustments are made in the position of the arms, there is a surprisingly long period that the arms will continue to stay up. In a way, this may be a symbolic foretaste of the ascent from point-eight to point-nine where intention plays the dominant role.

When a person has experienced the level of health corresponding to point-eight for many consecutive years or decades, it can be heartbreaking to lose it, for example, in a serious accident. But when one has lived at a healthy level for a long time, even a catastrophe may not be irreversible. Thus in every generation we seem to hear stories of accident victims who were told they would never walk again, and yet devote themselves totally, using every quantum of their will, strength, and persistence until they achieve their goal and return to quasi-normal functioning. It is as though there is an overwhelming instinct hard-wired into our DNA to regain this state of health and normal function if we lose it. It must be intimately tied to our survival as individuals and as a species. In other words, the force of healing can manifest a power vastly greater than our ordinary conception of it or even our trust in it. It is only our thinking and our beliefs that put limits on it, and constrict its potential.

This latter possibility (of accidentally losing one's health) underlines another quality of point-eight in the healing octave, and that is, even at this stage, one's health can be lost. Though it represents a relatively stable state, point-eight is more like a beautiful grassy meadow below the last pitch up to the top of the peak. It is not yet the top of the mountain itself. And to carry the analogy a bit further, one can figuratively "fall asleep" even in this high place, wander over to the edge of the meadow and fall off a cliff, just as it can happen at any other point on the circle.

However, if one "loses it" at point-seven, as we have seen, the descent can take them all the way back to point-one. It would seem that the fall from point-eight, however, would land one only at point-five, in accordance with the 8→5 inner line. In other words, someone in a stable state of health who becomes ill, would slide backward just to point-five, a place of only slight dysfunction. And this does happen some of the time, but we know that extreme health challenges can occur even to people in a high state of aerobic and muscular conditioning. They seem to be vulnerable to certain diseases, serious accidents, and injuries like the rest of us, although perhaps not as frequently.

In my opinion, the 8→5 inner line has a positive as well as a negative aspect as do the other backward facing inner lines which are 4→2 and 7→1. We have discussed how at point-four if one is not making progress with their treatment or is unhappy with their doctor they will abandon that therapy and actually return to point-two to re-initiate the sub-process of deciding on some other kind of help. But 4→2 can also be a look backward to validate one's decision, and be a source of encouragement.

At point-seven, if one imagines they are healed and reverts to their old habits, they will find themselves starting completely over at point-one, as sick as they were the first time, which often happens to recovering addicts of various kinds, when they "fall off the wagon" after many months or years of sobriety.

The 7→1 inner line however, also has positive possibilities and these are:

1) a warning that one can heed, a premonition of the endpoint of either failing to continue in one's healing program or falling into complacency;

2) the inspiration gained by the contrast to point-one, that is, seeing how far one has come in their healing, feeling the satisfaction of that, and acquiring the motivation from that glimpse backward to aspire to regain a more sustainable and energetic level of health.

Remember, the inner lines are simply an opening that the universe has given to us, to be able to reconnect with another point in time—an earlier or later part of the process—as we reach each gravity-center of the octave. How we use that opening, that opportunity, is our choice depending upon many factors.

So these openings, specifically the ones at 4→2, 7→1, and 8→5 can literally pull us backward to repeat a part of the process due to unfortunate choices, unforeseen consequences of our actions, or a lack of awareness. In all these cases ( 4→2, 7→1, and 8→5) if one falls backward and must repeat part of the process, we can conclude, in retrospect, that there must have been an insurmountable obstacle to going forward.

The positive aspect of the 8→5 inner line is analogous to its counterpart on the right side of the circle, the 1→4 inner line. At point-one, when one is suffering with their problem enough to finally acknowledge the need for help, there is a clairvoyant moment of seeing ahead—a visualizing of oneself receiving exactly the treatment that is needed, and this vision facilitates the journey to point-two and beyond.

At point-eight, one looks back to point-five to re-assess and to revisit the progress one has made, and in some cases learn how it could have been quicker, more direct, with fewer set-backs, and also to recall what worked and what energized the healing. We learn from pondering our mistakes, and we learn from appreciating our successes. This is another aspect of the 8→5 inner line.

Finding oneself at point-eight seems to be a time to recapitulate an earlier part of the process and coincidentally, or lawfully, the writer finds himself engaged in that act in the previous few paragraphs of this chapter.

An example of the 8→5 look-backward happened in my life several years ago: During a period of stable health, seemingly out of nowhere, a vivid memory suddenly appeared from many years earlier, after I had been in the hospital for another uncontrollable asthma attack in the spring of 1972 in Boston. When I recovered, my wife came to pick me up from the hospital, and as we were driving through the outer edges of the downtown area, I was overwhelmed by a desire for calorie-rich decadent food. This impulse arose after three days of eating small portions of hospital food that was so processed and bland it made school cafeteria lunches seem upscale. Three days of that deficient diet caused me to be ravenous. So on an impulse we stopped at one of those blue-collar sandwich shops that were abundant in Boston in those days, and I bought a large roast beef sandwich on a bun with all the "fixings" and a chocolate milkshake, for the long ride home in the car. Of course that kind of food is not the wisest choice for a person recovering from an illness, barely reaching point-five. I remembered even as I was eating, feeling ambivalent about that rich (and what I understand now as inflammation-promoting) food.

So, what was the function of that memory? And why did it pop into my head when it did? These are questions that are not yet totally resolved, but in general I think that the 8→5 inner line in this case relates to "repairing the past." In other words, it is a change I can make in myself now, in response to the re-experiencing of an old event, so that I (and maybe others?) won't have to repeat these kinds of mistakes in the future.

In this sense point-eight is an ideal place where the saying of Jane Heap: "Repair the past, Prepare the future," can come to fruition.

Another view of point-eight can be seen by analogy to its place in the octave of the transformation of food by the body, described in the chapter Purgatory of *Beelzebub's Tales*. In the "food octave," point-eight represents the fine substance, Exioëhary, which is concentrated in the male and female sex organs. This "substance" represents the mysterious energy that gives sperm and ova an independent life, that is, a life separate and distinct from the organism that created them. From any perspective this is another of the great miracles of our world—that basic digested nutrients can be assembled and transformed to produce living cells capable of reproducing themselves into a new organism. For several hundred million years, this process has been so universal and so reliable that now we take it completely for granted.

According to Gurdjieff, Exioehary embodies the highest or finest energy resulting from the digestion and transformation of the food we eat.

Also, as we are learning, a further miracle is that Exioehary can be used not only for reproduction, but for both creativity and personal evolution, which represents going beyond point-eight. An example that encompasses both is the effort to remember oneself. It is both a Work effort and a creative effort, because the reminding factor that enabled this self-aware state the previous time, probably won't work the next time; it is not an experience that can be repeated automatically. The energy for this creative effort is the fine energy produced at point-eight of the octave of the transformation of our ingested food. (See Figure Ap-4 on page 119 for the complete enneagram of the "Food Octave.")

When people squander a critical mass of the precursor of this energy at point-seven, through negative imagination, daydreams, and fantasies, there will be an insufficient amount to go beyond point-eight, or perhaps even to reach point-eight, in terms of being able to express their creativity or obtain results from inner work.

The question in practical terms (in the octave of self-development) is, am I willing to sacrifice my fantasies, daydreams, and indulgence in energy-wasting emotional reactions, so that there will be enough of this fine energy left for creative expression and in addition, to come in touch with a deeper reality?

Likewise, this stage of the healing octave is also a creative process, as is every step from the initial treatment (4→5 interval) onward, but more and more as we ascend the left side of the circle. The ability to reach point-eight also involves some sacrifice, as we noted in the previous chapter. In fact in most fields of life, there is space for a creative process only if one sacrifices their habitual activity.

So often in my practice, I encounter patients with a health problem that is totally one-of-a-kind. Because of their unique heredity, their idiosyncratic habits, because of perhaps unusual accidents or trauma that had peculiar cumulative effects, and because of all the individual ways that they have addressed these problems, they end up with complex conditions unique to them alone. For these patients, there is no recipe, no formula, no precedent described in any medical literature. Working to restore their health is a creative process, like an improvisational dance. Through continual feedback from these unusual patients after each method tried, we incorporate the techniques and remedies that work, reject the ones that don't work, and learn from clinical trial and error, until an effective treatment regimen is created. Also the patient may need to make certain changes in their lifestyle, in their attitude, and sacrifices of habitual activities that are hindering their healing.

Many of the techniques of Chiropractic developed in the last century were discovered by searching for better ways to help patients with unique or unusual problems, where all the standard methods failed, and something new was needed.

But even without the help of a doctor or therapist, patients often find amazing, unprecedented ways to help themselves, through trial and error, persistence, and serendipity.

One more thought that may be appropriate for this chapter, is the importance of realizing that there is a fundamental difference between the process of healing and most other processes.

Through healing, the organism is trying to restore a system that in the past functioned normally. Remember that for the first 30 or so years of life, most people enjoy various levels of normal health. When it fails for one reason or another, an irresistible healing impulse arises that attempts to restore the system to its previous level of health. When we lose our equilibrium, there is an imperative to focus upon regaining our balance.

In most other processes, on the other hand, one either starts with nothing but raw materials and ideas and creates something; or else starts with a potential, as in the learning of a skill or craft, and works to achieve some level of mastery.

The octave of spiritual development, however, like the octave of healing, is another exception to the way most processes unfold. There are aspects of restoration in the Work of bringing the mind back to a state where unnecessary suffering and unnecessary ego excesses have fallen away, allowing a simpler, quieter and more self-sincere approach to life. In the process of growing up in a socially dysfunctional culture, one acquires "baggage," analogous to contracting a disease, then has to Work on oneself in order to restore the essence of their child-like honesty and simplicity.

In healing, one also works to restore the system back to the normal functioning and energy it once had, although at point-eight this is a relative attainment; the energy level may never be as high as it was earlier in life. On the other hand, the 8→9 interval yields possibilities that go beyond restoration, as we shall see.

CHAPTER 10

# The 8→9 Interval, Point 9 and the Completion of the Octave

The way I have described point-eight, the reader may have acquired the impression that it is the culmination of the healing process. But point-eight simply represents the restoration of one's normal functioning. To go beyond point-eight is to actualize a state where one's health is even better and more robust than it was before the illness, injury, or other dysfunction began to manifest.

For example, after a fracture heals, the bone will sometimes be harder and denser at that site than it was before the trauma. This extra density after a fracture is usually related to the degree to which the recovering person uses the affected bone—the more use (that is, after the collagen framework has been re-established) the harder the bone will be. The extra use requires intention; it doesn't happen by itself.

In fact the central feature of the 8→9 interval, also called the Si-Do interval, is just this intention—to go beyond what would seem necessary for a recovery, to go "the extra mile" to insure that one is healthier, stronger and more resistant to stress, disease or injury than before the imbalance appeared at point-zero. In other words, completing the healing octave isn't simply a restoration of one's former state of health, but an intentional upgrading, as it were, to a higher state of functioning where there is more wholeness, in a physiological sense, and more balance in one's life than before the healing process began.

Before continuing with this section it is necessary to emphasize that I myself am entering a realm here that is somewhat removed from my own experience. So even though I can describe the target at point-nine from observation of those who have apparently reached a completion of the octave, the path to arrive there can only be inferred and understood in a partial way by those of us who have not experienced it personally. But it will still be useful to identify the known attributes and conceptual characteristics of this final part of the octave, so that at least those aspiring to an even higher level of health and wholeness will have some discreet touchstones along the way.

A central feature of the 8→9 interval, as I noted earlier, comes from the food octave described in the chapter Purgatory in *Beelzebub's Tales*. Gurdjieff is very vague about this particular step but gives one or two tantalizing morsels of information, which can be applied to the octave of healing as well. The first morsel is the name of the interval; "the intentionally-actualized Mdnel-in." Remember that the first shock point in the octave, the Mi-Fa interval, which passed through point-three, was called by Gurdjieff, the "mechano-coinciding Mdnel-in." "Mechano-coinciding" vs. "intentionally-actualized." Passing through point-three—where the effort is to come into contact with the help that is needed—is where one first interfaces with the outer world, which either happens to cooperate or else provide resistance. The patient's octave mechanically collides with or coincides with a much larger process and this interaction either allows the patient to reach point-four or not. But with the 8→9 interval, it is only the quality of one's intention that provides the shock to complete the octave.

I recall an example of this kind of intention from the words of the pioneering physical-fitness guru, Jack Lalane. When asked why he worked out in his home gym two hours every morning before breakfast (5 AM–7 AM) no matter how he felt or no matter what other obligations he had that day, his reply was, "I have a sacred obligation to my body."

That was the attitude that powered his intention. Perhaps that attitude was based on the belief that the body is the "temple of the spirit," the vessel that contains a sacred and mysterious force. Or perhaps he believed that the degree that one values their soul, or spiritual life, must equal the care that they direct towards optimizing their health and capability of the body.

Interestingly, there are very few religions or spiritual teachings in the Western tradition that put much emphasis in practice on perfect health, although they may value it theoretically.

Gurdjieff taught that personal evolution must be balanced among the development of the three centers: mental, emotional, and moving/instinctive. However Gurdjieff's movements, the sacred dances, speak more to the "brain" of the body than to health itself. (But it should be noted that without a level of health at least up to point-seven, it is very difficult to practice the movements.)

Gurdjieff's own health was ravaged by infectious diseases, bullet wounds, etc. during his extensive travels through dangerous territory in his quest to discover ancient spiritual secrets. Then it was ravaged again by a near-fatal auto accident in France in the 1920's. From my vantage point, it seems that he then sacrificed his healing and his health in order to complete the task of spreading his teaching and his understanding into the world. Unfortunately, some of his followers have imitated his habits of drinking and smoking rather than understanding his sacrifice for them—alcohol tranquilizes pain, nicotine helps clear the mind for intense efforts of concentration; and these followers ended up prematurely ruining their own health in turn.

However, the more I contemplate the complexities of the 8→9 interval, the more I see how multifaceted it can be. Nature brings us only to point-eight, a state where all of our parts are in relative working order, but where we haven't pushed far enough in any direction to go beyond our limits, or to have reached a place where we can become a finely-tuned instrument for some larger purpose.

One idea to remember is that the 8→9 interval, like all the others, represents another new direction that requires new kinds of efforts. The image that comes to mind in terms of this particular new direction is that of a leap. One may be skiing down a mountain having a certain kind of experience then hit a jump, and all of a sudden the skier is flying through the air—an entirely new kind of experience which requires a different kind of effort. Motorcycle jumpers take similar leaps. An example from the spiritual literature concerns the Yaqui master, Don Juan, who taught his pupil, Carlos Casteneda to take a leap and jump across the "abyss." The latter is not only an intentional act, but the outcome is unknown. Perhaps in the same way, point-nine is shrouded behind a figurative veil for the subject taking the leap beyond point-eight.

In one way of thinking, point-eight does represent a completion of the healing process—that is as far as nature can take us in a mechanical sense. Yet there is a possibility for humans to go beyond that point and take a leap into the unknown that leads to a higher completion. The difficulty here is to understand what this "higher completion" would be; that is, point-nine, which Gurdjieff calls "Resulzarion" in the food octave. (This is the other morsel of information that he gave us.)

In terms of the octave of spiritual development Resulzarion would perhaps represent the completing results of what Gurdjieff calls "being-Partkdolg-duty," that is, intentional efforts that use the special energy available at point-eight. But in the process of spiritual evolution there never really is a final completion. Every "result" can be a springboard for another challenge, another new process.

As we ascend from point-eight, it may be that there is a convergence between the octave of healing and the octave of spiritual evolution. That would imply that completion of the process of healing would also be an elusive concept to pin down. In other words, point-nine of the healing octave may be a dynamic fluid state rather than an end point.

If we take into account the inevitable aging process, the unstoppable passage of time, unforeseen crises, etc., there are always new challenges for the human organism. There are new challenges, and perhaps narrower, more contracted limits to go beyond. Then there is the complicating issue that healing must also occur, as we saw for the 7→8 interval, on an emotional and psychological level. To ascend beyond point-eight one may need to transcend even a healthy ego. It is in this way that healing and inner work begin to converge.

This brings us to another ingredient in the formula that allows one to complete either octave, and that is the impulse of love. Intention, as I have discussed, is essential at this final step. But intention alone, and will alone, are not sufficient to complete the octave because lawfully they provoke resistance. The more one wills oneself to complete a project, the more stubborn the resistance. Many octaves are never completed. People build houses and move into them before they are finished, authors write novels and either don't complete them or fail to see them published, artists let paintings languish in their studios unfinished or unframed, etc. In my experience, love is the third force in this final step of the octave that allows the process to come to completion—the love of the process, the love of the work.

I realized this about six years ago when I was building a large, floor-to-ceiling stone hearth behind my wood stove. There was the usual resistance to completing the process, as there always is, and I easily could have given into it and called it "good enough" at two or three different points near the end. But it was my love of working with the stones (which was also an arena for working on myself) that enabled me to complete the project. I had a vision for how it would look, I loved to see how each stone fit in the borders and I really wished to see the finished product.

Of course, I have completed a few other projects in my life, but this was the first time that I was conscious of going through an 8→9 interval, aware of the tremendous resistance, and able to witness that simply being determined to complete it was necessary but not sufficient. It took a gentle force from my heart to melt the resistance. This actually was one of the more memorable experiences of my life, observing myself complete that project.

This latter experience can inform people wishing to ascend from point-eight that have an intention to embark upon a discipline to go beyond their normal level of health. Many people are determined and understand the need, but the resistance given by their lives becomes overwhelming. However there is that minority of people who love how it feels when they are "in shape" and when their bodies are moving, and when they are able to perform their skill or craft at the highest level. It is the love of the process that may be able to take them all the way to point-nine.

The emotional force that is needed at the 8→9 interval is not a love of the body nor a narcissistic self-love, but again, a love of the process. Ideally, it has the possibility of being a love of life itself. It is the relationship between me and the universe. The Japanese have a term for this kind of relationship; they call it Cho-Wa. If there is an inner state that would characterize point-nine in the healing octave, I would speculate that it would be something like Cho-Wa. This latter term is defined as a state of inner harmony or a state like being in love, where there is a quickening of the life-force, a heightening of perceptions, an opening of the heart, and a compassionate attention continually bathing the object of one's love, which in this case can be everything. Of course, this is a state that, as I am, I have only fleeting moments of feeling this way—but enough to know that it is possible. Also, note that the state of Cho-Wa represents a relationship with the outer world; it is not simply a higher state of health described in terms of one's organic functioning. This is another difference between point-eight and point-nine. In this sense, one change of direction in the 8→9 interval is a transition from a self-centered attitude to a movement outward. In Dr. Bach's words,

> As there is one great root cause of disease—namely self-love, so there is one great certain method of relief of all suffering, the conversion of self-love into devotion to others. [1]

In my understanding, self-love, a term Gurdjieff has also used to describe one of our major obstacles, is not really love at all, strictly speaking, but part of the grip of ego which engenders varying degrees of fear, and isolation from other people. For example, vanity is an obsession with how I appear to others which can only be based upon internal considering and fear, not a real caring for oneself. Narcissism, too is a neurotic fascination with one's surface features that has almost nothing to do with real love.

Therefore, we might conclude that a necessary part of the effort to reach point-nine is to overcome our slavery to the ego—to put a love of others before our imagined fears. In Gurdjieff's words, "to put my neighbor's welfare above my own." Obviously, this is easier said than done, which is one reason so few people attain to this level.

If Dr. Bach is correct, disease begins in the soul; or in more clinical terms, disease begins with emotional and/or psychological imbalances, of which there is a long list that we are all familiar with. So if the subject can bring this higher part of themselves into balance, in theory the body will be able to follow suit.

---

1 Bach, *Heal Thyself* (p 19).

There appears to be a great paradox here: when all my attention is focused only upon myself and my own well-being, it actually limits my progress. When this is the case, the octave can proceed to point-eight, maybe a bit beyond, but then the energy turns in on itself so to speak, and begins some kind of involution. In order to attain point-nine and complete the process a corresponding amount of energy needs to go outward; there needs to be an exchange. And the energy we offer outward seems to come back to us tenfold.

From the Taoist tradition, a similar idea was expressed by my Chi Gong teacher in Beijing, Wan Su Jian. He conveyed his understanding that when one limits oneself to self-healing techniques, progress is slow; but when one engages in service to others, progress is greatly accelerated. I have verified this dichotomy for myself. When I teach Chi Gong or other aspects of self-healing or lead meditation groups, it helps me in many ways:

1) It enables me to adhere more faithfully to my own practice discipline and bring it to a higher level,

2) It forces me to formulate for my students what I actually understand and shows me where my understanding is lacking,

3) It encourages me to "practice what I preach" about healing and health choices, and finally,

4) When I make these efforts to reach out to others, it seems to attract energy from some inexhaustible source, energy that seems to help everyone in the group and is not available when I am self-absorbed.

Another example of the kind of intentional service that would facilitate the 8→9 journey would be to simply offer one's expertise to those who are struggling at a lower point on the healing octave. The receivers of this expertise can draw inspiration, courage, and energy from someone who has "been through it." For example, survivors of cancer and other diseases can be invaluable leaders of support groups for people struggling to reach point-five or even to find point-four, and in turn this service may help these facilitators to complete their own octave. Likewise, ex-addicts are often the most credible mentors to those "bottoming out" and lost in their addiction. Service to others in almost any healing situation helps the server in many ways.

Sometime around 2000, Master Wan and a few of his older students traveled to remote Western China to offer their assistance at a large orphanage housing over 600 children. These children had been brought there from all over China and were either autistic, brain-damaged, or otherwise severely developmentally disabled. They were essentially castaways. Medical attention at the institution was lacking, and the overall morale was very low. Master Wan and his students spent weeks there attending to all the details of hygiene, sanitation, nutrition, etc., and he personally examined each child, assessing their overwhelming needs. It was a task that was daunting and next to impossible, given the severe defects of the children and the limited resources available. But Master Wan did what he could medically and with his Chi, and finally to lift their spirits he taught the older ones—a group of about 40-50 orphans—a song, their own song. They practiced it every day, and after they learned it, a short video was filmed by one of Master Wan's students of their performance. The words that these special children sang, in a paraphrased translation from my memory was as follows:

> "We are like rocks buried under the ground.
> May our faith and our perseverance lift us up to the surface,
> so that together we may form a string of stepping stones,
> and when people walk on us,
> may our path lead them to happiness and fulfillment."

Not only was this a creative, life-altering experience for the children and staff at the orphanage, it was a very emotional experience for those of us who saw the film and even for those who heard about it second-hand.

I am certain that this quality of intentional service helped bring Master Wan closer to point-nine in his own octave of self-mastery because, as Gurdjieff appreciated, the heart needs to develop as well as the body and the mind.

In relation to completing the octave of healing and the octave of inner work, which as I mentioned, converge somewhat at this final step, there are questions that remain. For example, is there actually a discrete point at which, as for the other gravity-centers, we can say, "this experience marks the arrival at point-nine?" Is it when an initiate reaches a stage when they totally devote themselves to other people, like Mother Teresa, or the Dalai Lama, or the historical saints and gurus? Must there be a functioning at a higher level of consciousness that is not available to us mortals? And is a mastery of the body a necessary part of the completion of the healing octave? Two examples of people who combined mastery of the body with a dedication to higher service are:

1) the legendary Apache holy-man, Stalking Wolf, who was the teacher of Tom Brown[2], and

2) the 142 year old Taoist martial-arts master described by his student.[3]

Both of these men were in perfect health until virtually the end of their lives, and were capable of physical skills, stamina, and a harmonious relationship with their surroundings that far surpassed anything of which I had ever conceived.

There is an ancient Japanese martial art described by Glenn Morris.[4] Dr. Morris learned that in this particular tradition, to be awarded a fifth-degree black belt, the initiate not only had to master the whole body of knowledge and technique in that lineage, but he had to create something new: a new exercise, a new technique, a new movement—something of his own added to the repertoire of the lineage. This final task embodies the intention, the creativity, the love of the Work, and the service to others that are the hallmarks of the journey from point-eight to point-nine.

Another question is whether the healing octave can be considered complete when only the one part of the body that was injured or ill is again brought into balance with the whole? Are there perhaps many small octaves that together coalesce into this picture of a great healing enneagram that I have visualized and presented here?

As we approach what is just beyond the horizon there are more questions than answers. Maybe it is best to leave it that way rather than try to intuit or conjure up the most plausible conclusion, like the way I used to approach exams in college. For this reason, point-nine, even though I can understand it theoretically as a point of completion, of balance, of wholeness, and perhaps of mastery—as an experience it will remain a little out of reach, a bit beyond my ability to describe it from my own practical reference point at this moment in time.

2 Brown, *Grandfather*.
3 Deng Ming Tao, *The Wandering Taoist*.
4 Morris, *Path Notes of an American Ninja Master*.

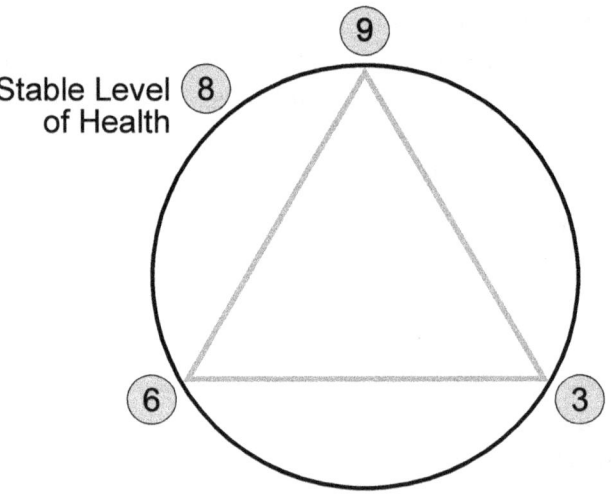

**Figure 10-1,** *Partial enneagram focusing on the 8→9 Interval*

The 8→9 interval (also called the "intentionally actualized mdnel-in") is the completing step of the healing octave, and can be thought of as an optional step that brings one's health to a higher and more vibrant level.

## Appendix
# Complete Enneagram Symbols

On the following pages are the complete enneagrams of the processes discussed in the chapters including:

1) *Enneagram of Healing*, which of course is the subject of the book.

2) *Enneagram of Spiritual Development*, which was found to have many similarities to the enneagram of healing,

3) *Enneagram of the Lord's Prayer*, whose relationship to the process of healing was an accidental discovery by the author, and

4) *Enneagram of the Food Octave*, which is described (without actual reference to the enneagram itself) in the chapter Purgatory, of *Beelzebub's Tales*, and has been a reference point for the understanding of octaves and enneagrammatic processes in general for many students of the Gurdjieff teaching, for at least 33 years.

The enneagram diagrams shown in this appendix, as in most other books on the subject, traditionally have the nine points labeled with the words that best describe that step of the process. Keep in mind that for the first two enneagrams shown here, the words I have chosen to denote each point are only approximations—limited by language itself—and that there may be other words that are equivalent or even more accurate.

Also, in addition to the nine points, I might well have labeled the intervals and the inner lines if there were more space on the symbol. However, at least for the enneagram of healing, these are described in the chapters.[1]

---

[1] See also Steffan Soule's book, *Accomplish the Impossible*, which identifies and names the inner lines for many different enneagrams. His interpretation of the significance of some inner lines agrees with mine, and for other inner lines, our two interpretations lead to further questions.

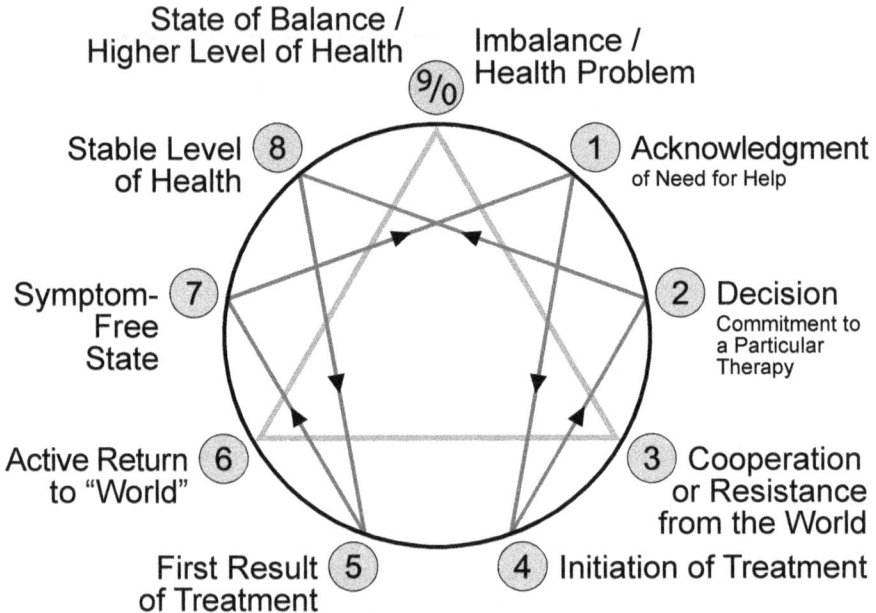

**Figure Ap-1,** *Enneagram of Healing*

The complete enneagram showing the essential experience or landmark at each point of the process. The intervals and inner lines are discussed in the individual chapters.

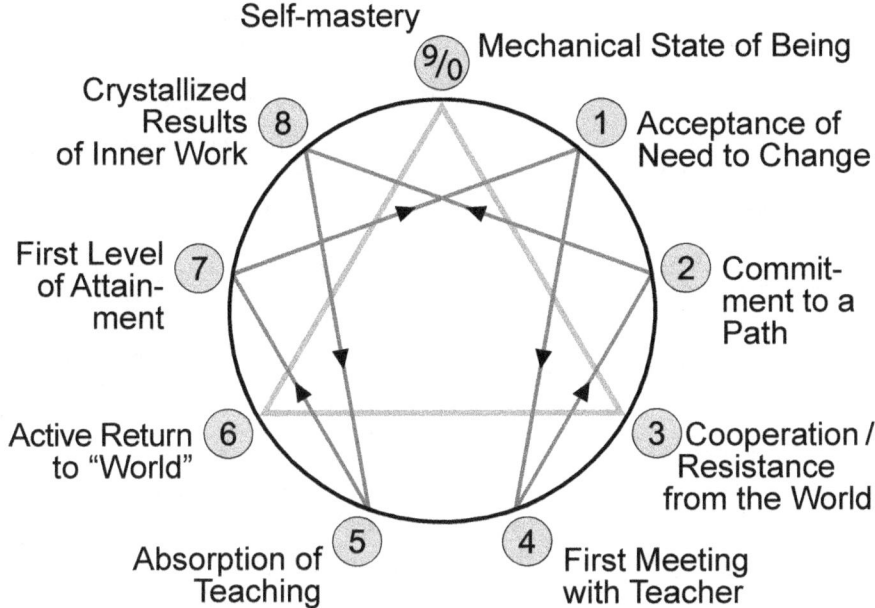

**Figure Ap-2,** *Enneagram of Spiritual Development*

The complete enneagram showing the essential experience or landmark at each point. Some of these points as well as the intervals between them are discussed in the text, especially when there is a close analogy to the healing enneagram.

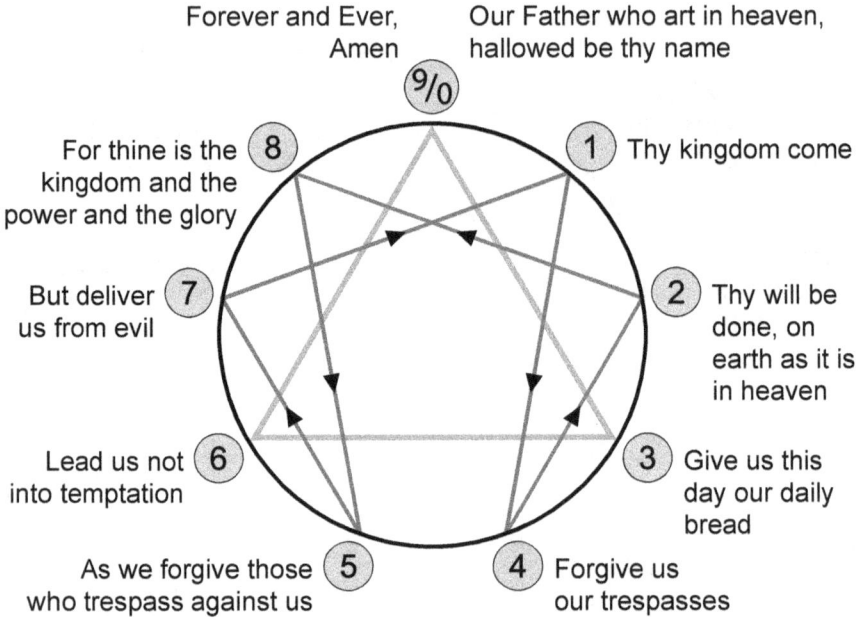

**Figure Ap-3,** *Enneagram of the Lord's Prayer*

> In this interpretation, "Our Father. . ." would be placed at point-zero, and can be thought of as the state of the universe at the onset of creation, that is, at the beginning. The final phrase, "forever and ever, amen," is placed at point-nine, and can be considered as a culmination. There is no discrete ending or completion of this octave, instead a limitless eternity.
>
> For different interpretations of the Lord's Prayer enneagram, see Anthony Blake's book, *The Intelligent Enneagram* or John Bennett's book, *Enneagram Studies*.

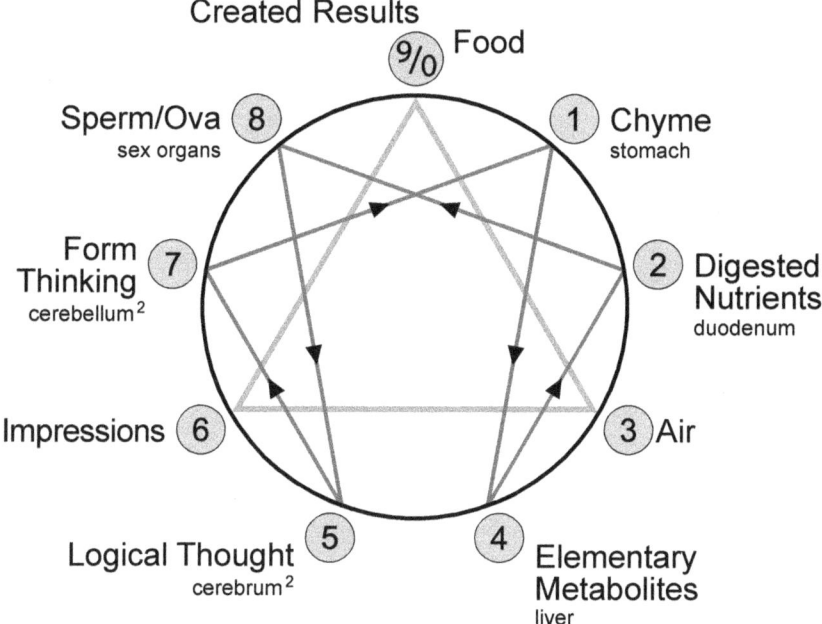

**Figure Ap-4,** *Enneagram of the Transformation of Food*

> In essence, the points in this enneagram actually represent the energy or vibrational level associated with each substance listed around the circle, which become finer as the process continues. The 4→5 interval in this octave denotes the transformation of metabolic energy into thought/brain activity which is one of the great miracles of life. Another miraculous phenomenon is that sex energy (embodied in the germ cells) can be used for creativity or inner work. The Gurdjieffian terms for the gravity-centers are: point-one, being-protoehary; point-two, being-defteroehary; point-four, being-tritoehary; point-five, being-tetarteohary; point-seven, being-piandjiohary; point-eight, being-exioëhary; point-nine, resulzarion.

---

[2] In contemporary terms, cerebrum would perhaps be frontal cortex, and cerebellum would be parietal cortex.

# Acknowledgments

The octave of my relationship to the enneagram had its origins almost forty years ago after reading *In Search of the Miraculous*. During the succeeding decades there were many, many people toward whom I now feel grateful, who stimulated my interest in this subject through the purity of their own quest. They inspired me with their insights and their being, and helped to create conditions where my study could bear fruit. A very few of those, both friends and teachers, were Elizabeth Van Renen, Alan Joel, Kamori Cattadoris, Barrett McMaugh, Mrs. Annie Lou Staveley, Tom Shiolas, Beverly Viers, Michael Smyth, Will Mesa, Dr. Keith Buzzell, Dr. John Lester and Cari Kimler. Of course there were many others through the years who helped further my understanding of the enneagram, some through personal contact, and some through their writings. I am grateful to all of those not mentioned here by name for their devotion toward understanding cosmic laws and the workings of the universe, which has been a continuing source of inspiration for me.

There were also all the doctors, healers, and health practitioners over the years who contributed in both practical and theoretical ways to my understanding and well-being, including those mentioned in the text, for whom I have a very deep gratitude.

The Do for this book was sounded in December 2010 when I gave a talk on the enneagram of healing to the Metanoia Society of Bend, Oregon. Thanks to all those present that evening, and again one year later, for their enthusiastic response, which gave me energy to continue with this project.

The physical book itself was made possible through the intentional service of Steffan Soule, who devoted so many hours to transforming it from a manuscript/word document into a form ready to be printed, through his wizardry with the Adobe computer programs. His contribution was essential and is greatly appreciated. Thanks also to our wives, Barbara Halliday and Winnie Givot, for enduring countless hours listening to us editing and putting the book together, and also for their suggestions and help with various questions as they arose, and thanks to Winnie for her fine portrait of me on the back cover.

Thanks also to Catherine Knemeyer for typing the first draft of the manuscript into a word processing document during the spring and summer of 2011, to Toddy Smyth for her thoughtful suggestions, and to Darcy Sinclair for her ideas about the design of the front cover. And finally, thanks to the doctor, whose name I have long-forgotten and was unable to re-discover, who brought back a photo of the ancient line-drawing from Taiwan, shown on the front cover.

# Bibliography

The books listed here are the ones that appear in the footnotes in the text. In addition there are included a few general references on related material.

Bach, Edward. *Heal Thyself.* First published by C.W. Daniel, 1931; Random House edition, 2004.

Bennett, John.
*Enneagram Studies.* Samuel Weiser, 1983.
*Talks on Beelzebub's Tales.* Samuel Weiser, 1988.

Blake, A.G.E. *The Intelligent Enneagram.* Shambala, 1996.

Brown, Tom. *Grandfather.* Berkley, 1996, 2001.

Buzzell, Keith A. *Perspectives on Beelzebub's Tales.* Fifth Press, 2005.

Deng Ming-Dao. *The Wandering Taoist.* Harper and Row, 1983.

Givot, Irv.
*Seven Aspects of Self Observation.* Two Rivers Press, 1998.
*Healing in China.* Xlibris, 2004.

Gurdjieff, George.
*Beelzebub's Tales to his Grandson.* Harcourt Brace and Co., 1950; Two Rivers Press edition, 1993.
*Meetings with Remarkable Men.* Routledge, 1963; E.P. Dutton edition, 1969.

Gurdjieff, George. *Life is Real Only Then, When "I Am"*. Triangle Editions, 1975.

Morris, Glenn. *Path Notes of an American Ninja Master*. North Atlantic Books, 1993.

Nicoll, Maurice. *Psychological Commentaries on the Teachings Of Gurdjieff and Ouspensky, vol.2*. Vincent Stuart, 1952; Stuart and Watkins edition, 1970.

Ouspensky, P.D. *In Search of the Miraculous*. Harcourt Brace Jovanovich, 1949, 1977.

Palmer, Helen. *The Enneagram*. Harper, 1991.

Pollan, Michael.
*The Omnivore's Dilemma*. Penguin Press, 2006.
*In Defense of Food*. Penguin Press, 2008.

Rawicz, Slawomir (and Ronald Dowling). *The Long Walk*. Lyons Press, 1997, 2006.

Soule, Steffan. *Accomplish the Impossible*. ATOM Press, 2011.

Staveley, A.L. *Themes*. Two Rivers Press, 1981.

Weeks, Nora. *The Medical Discoveries of Edward Bach*. Physician. C.W. Daniel, 1940, 2007.

# Index

1→4 inner line  9, 19-21, 25, 102
2→8 inner line  9, 24-26, 35, 70, 94
4→2 inner line  9, 40, 55, 101-102
5→7 inner line  9, 55, 61, 67, 70-71, 74
7→1 inner line  9, 74, 76, 80, 93, 101-102
8→5 inner line  9, 101-103

0→1 interval  16-17, 25, 29, 35
1→2 interval  18, 20-23, 25, 29, 35
2→(3)→4 interval  20, 29-30
4→5 interval  40, 46-51, 53-55, 57, 65, 92, 104, 121
5→(6)→7 interval  57, 61, 62, 65, 78
7→8 interval  77, 85-88, 90, 92, 94-95, 110
8→9 interval  88, 105, 107-109, 111-113, 116

2→4→2 cycle  40
5→7→1 triad  71-72

point-zero  15-17, 107, 120
point-one  9, 15-21, 23, 32, 39, 60, 71, 74, 76, 78-79, 93, 98, 100-102, 121
point-two  18-19, 21, 23-24, 26, 29, 32, 40, 70, 94, 98, 101-102, 121
point-three  11, 29-31, 34-35, 62, 67, 98, 108
point-four  18, 20, 23, 31, 33-36, 39-46, 49-50, 57, 80, 82, 98, 101, 108, 113, 121
point-five  33, 39, 41-42, 49-50, 54, 57-65, 70-72, 76-77, 79-80, 82, 98-102, 113, 121
point-six  11, 30, 61, 62, 66-69, 80
point-seven  41, 50, 55, 60-61, 64-66, 69-70, 72, 75-78, 80, 83, 85-86, 88, 91-94, 99-101, 103, 109, 121
point-eight  22, 50, 61, 77-79, 85-86, 88-89, 91-95, 97, 99-100, 102-105, 107, 109-113, 115, 121
point-nine  11, 30, 100, 108, 110-115, 120-121

Armstrong, Lance  59-60
asthma  18, 32-34, 46, 102

Bach, Dr. Edward  51-52, 81, 93, 112
*Beelzebub's Tales*  19, 22, 63-64, 78-79, 88, 103, 108, 117
being-Partkdolg-duty  110
Belcultassi  19, 21
Bennett, John  47, 64, 100, 120
Binder, Dr. Tim  45-46
blind men and the elephant dilemma  14
Brown, Tom  45, 115
Buddhist  16, 41

Casteneda, Carlos  44, 110
cerebellum  79, 121
Chakdud Tulku Rinpoche  41
Chi  90-91, 113-114
Chiropractic  24, 31, 36, 45-46, 61, 65, 76, 104
Chiropractor  45, 58-60
Cho-Wa  111-112

deflections  7
de Salzmann, Jeanne  43-44, 46
discernment  23, 40, 48-49
disharmonizing  62-63
disharmonizing mdnel-in  62
Don Juan  45, 109
downhill octave  80

effort to remember oneself  103
enhanced openness  43
enneagram  3-14, 16, 18, 24-25, 30, 34, 37, 39, 43, 47, 49-50, 54, 57-58, 60-61, 63-64, 67-68, 70, 74, 80, 88, 91, 93, 95, 98, 103, 115-121
Enneagram of Healing (figure)  118
Enneagram of Spiritual Development  117, 119
enneagram of the kitchen at work  47

Enneagram of the Lord's Prayer  120
Enneagram of the Transformation of Food  121
exioëhary  103, 121

faith  35, 70, 114
First Obligolnian Striving  22
Flower Remedies  51
food octave  79, 103, 108, 110
forgiveness  80-82, 85

gravity-center  7-8, 12, 68, 101
Gurdjieff, George  4, 8, 10, 17, 19, 22, 30, 34, 43-44, 46, 63, 69, 70, 78, 79, 86-88, 94, 103, 108-110, 112, 114
Harnel-Aoot  62-66, 70, 74
healing crisis  48-49, 92
healing influences  6
healing octave  8, 11, 17, 19, 22, 31, 34, 42, 47, 62, 67, 68, 70, 80-81, 83, 88, 98, 100, 104, 107, 110-111, 113, 115-116
Heap, Jane  103
help me, don't help me syndrome  39
homeostasis  97
hope  21, 35, 57, 65, 81, 85

imbalance  6, 15, 22, 107
inner lines  5, 8-9, 13, 20, 54, 74, 93, 101, 117-118
inner work  104, 110, 114, 121
intention  29, 40-41, 69, 73, 88, 91, 94, 100, 107-108, 110-111, 115
intentionally-actualized Mdnel-in  108
intentional service  113-114
intervals  8, 20, 58, 117-119
involution  113

Lalane, Jack  108
Law of Seven  10
Law of Three  10
Lord's Prayer  80, 117, 120

love (as an aspect of healing)  110-111

mdnel-in  10, 30, 62, 88, 116
mechano-coinciding  34, 108
Mechano-coinciding mdnel-in  30
Meetings With Remarkable Men  43
mi-fa interval  30, 35, 63
Morris, Dr. Glenn  115
musical octave  12-13, 58, 63-64

natural medicine  4

obstacle(s)  5-6, 16-17, 21, 24, 35, 50, 78, 82, 92, 94, 102, 112
octave of spiritual development  47, 86, 105, 110

parasympathetic nervous system  52
passive do  15
passivity  50-51
piandjoehary  78-79
Pollan, Michael  77
Prince Lubachevsky  69-70
Purgatory (Chapter of *Beelzebub's Tales*)  78, 103, 108, 117

Qi  12, 90
Qi Gong  90

relaxation  35-36, 52, 54
repairing the past  103
restoration  75, 105, 107
Resulzarion  110

self-mastery  18-19, 114
shock-point(s)  10, 31
Si-Do interval  107
sol-la interval  61, 63
Soule, Steffan  117

Spencer, Dr. Jeff  59
spirit patients  42
stability  97
Stalking Wolf  45, 115
Staveley, Mrs. Annie Lou  22, 88
stopinder(s)  8, 25, 30, 55, 62-63, 74, 85, 95
sub-clinical  75
submission  39, 47, 49-50
subtle energies  71
surgery  26, 49-50
sympathetic nervous system  52

Taoist  113, 115
Tetartoehary  79
*The Long Walk*  99
third force  111
Two Rivers Farm  17, 36, 43, 72

Wan Su Jian, Dr./Master  90, 113
Work (on oneself)  4, 18-19, 36, 43-44, 81, 87, 89, 92, 95, 103, 105, 115

www.ingramcontent.com/pod-product-compliance
Lightning Source LLC
Chambersburg PA
CBHW022136080426
42734CB00006B/382